REFUGEE CHILDREN

The Johns Hopkins Series in Contemporary Medicine and Public Health

Refugee Children

THEORY, RESEARCH, AND SERVICES

Edited by

Frederick L. Ahearn, Jr.

and

Jean L. Athey

THE JOHNS HOPKINS UNIVERSITY PRESS
Baltimore and London

© 1991 The Johns Hopkins University Press
All rights reserved
Printed in the United States of America

The Johns Hopkins University Press
701 West 40th Street
Baltimore, Maryland 21211-2190
The Johns Hopkins Press Ltd., London

The paper used in this book meets the minimum requirements
of American National Standards for Information Sciences—
Permanence of Paper for Printed Library Materials,
ANSI Z39.48-1984.

Library of Congress Cataloging-in-Publication Data

Refugee children : theory, research, and services / edited by
Frederick L. Ahearn, Jr. and Jean L. Athey.
    p.   cm. — (The Johns Hopkins series in contemporary medicine
and public health)
  Includes bibliographical references and index.
  ISBN 0-8018-4160-7
  1. Refugee children—Mental health—United States. 2. Refugee
children—Mental health services—United States. I. Ahearn,
Frederick L. II. Athey, Jean L., 1945– . III. Series.
RJ507.R44R44   1991
618.92'89'008694—dc20   90-25554

Contents

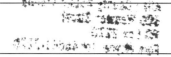

List of Contributors

John W. Berry, Ph.D., Professor, Department of Psychology, Queens University, Kingston, Ontario, Canada

Conchita M. Espino, Ph.D., clinical psychologist, Washington, D.C.

J. David Kinzie, M.D., Professor, Department of Psychiatry, Health Sciences University, Portland, Oregon

Jill E. Korbin, Ph.D., Associate Professor and Acting Chair, Department of Anthropology, Case Western Reserve University, Cleveland, Ohio

Margaret Leiper de Monchy, Coordinator, Refugee Assistance, Massachusetts Department of Mental Health, Boston, Massachusetts

Timothy Ready, Ph.D., Staff Associate, Division of Minority Health, Disease Prevention/Health Promotion, Association of American Medical Colleges, Washington, D.C.

Rubén G. Rumbaut, Ph.D., Professor, Department of Sociology, San Diego State University, San Diego, California

William Sack, M.D., Professor, Department of Psychiatry, Health Sciences University, Portland, Oregon

Joseph Westermeyer, M.D., M.P.H., Ph.D., Chairman, Department of Psychiatry, University of Oklahoma, Health Sciences Center, Oklahoma City, Oklahoma

Carolyn L. Williams, Ph.D., Associate Professor, Department of Public Health, University of Minnesota, Minneapolis, Minnesota

Acknowledgments

Many people and organizations have contributed to the success of this project. The Conference on Refugee Children Traumatized by War and Violence, which was held in Washington, D.C., in September 1988, initially focused attention on this subject. This conference was funded by the National Institute of Mental Health (NIMH) and the Maternal and Child Health Bureau in collaboration with Georgetown University Child Development Center and the National Catholic School of Social Service, Catholic University of America. The conference brought together a diverse group of researchers, service providers, and policy makers and provided them with the opportunity to share the data, information, and experience they had with child refugees. This book originated with that conference. Persons critical to the planning of the conference included Marva Benjamin, M.S.W., Georgetown University Child Development Center; Michael Fishman, M.D., and Jane Lin-Fu, Maternal and Child Health Bureau; Judith Katz-Leavy, M.Ed., and Ira Lourie, M.D., Child and Family Support Branch, NIMH; Richard Cravens, Ph.D., and Thomas Bornemann, Ed.D., Office of Refugee Mental Health, NIMH; and Elena Cohen, M.S.W., National Catholic School of Social Service, Catholic University of America.

We would also like to thank Janet Rosenkrantz, who assisted in typing chapters and bibliographies, and Kathy Curran and Jane Myers, for their expert technical editing.

We are most appreciative to each of these individuals and organizations. Without their support and assistance this book would not have been possible.

This book was co-edited by Dr. Athey in her private capacity. No official support or endorsement by the U.S. Public Health Service is intended or should be inferred.

Introduction

The United States Committee for Refugees (1990) reported that the number of the world's refugees increased 52.5 percent between 1984 and 1989, to an estimated 15.1 million displaced persons. Children represent nearly one-half of the total, or about 7.5 million (Office of the United Nations High Commissioner for Refugees, 1988).

This book explores typical experiences that identify the special physical, social, and mental health needs of refugee children, particularly those who have fled countries in which war or other forms of violence are widespread. The objectives of the book are three: (1) through the presentation of theory, research, and services to further delineate the effects on children of premigration, transmigration, and postmigration experiences; (2) to focus attention on and increase the understanding of child refugees; and (3) to explore issues in the delivery of services to such children and to describe model strategies for programing.

War, violence, economic deprivation, religious persecution, famine, and the hardships of flight make children particularly vulnerable to physical, social, and emotional traumas. Death of parents and loved ones, loss of home and destruction of community, separation, torture, and starvation are often the experiences of refugee children. The purpose of this book is to explore the implications of these traumas and propose interventions to assist this vulnerable population quickly and effectively.

In addition to extended deprivation and severe losses, refugee children also face the extraordinary requirements to adapt to a new and strange land. While a considerable literature exists concerning adult refugees, little has been published describing the special needs of children. And yet, children's needs are different from those of adults. Their development may be hampered when they depend on adults who themselves are in crisis, or they may acquire new roles because their parent or relative is not able to assume it. We know little about how children understand these events and how they are affected by them. For instance, how do refugee children manifest post-traumatic stress, grief, anxiety, and depression?

We hope that this volume begins to answer some important questions. How do children react to a refugee experience? What are their specific developmental, health, and mental health problems? What are their ways of adapting and coping? What types of intervention seem to offer promise for facilitating adaptation? Answers to these questions are important to a number of individuals: policy makers, who fashion our immigration laws; researchers, who need to continue to investigate how refugee children react to and cope with these traumas; and practitioners (psychologists, psychiatrists, social workers, nurses, clergy, and counselors), who must design and deliver the services for emotional support to assist this group.

REFERENCES

Office of the United Nations High Commissioner for Refugees (1988). Guidelines on refugee children. Interoffice memorandum no. 91/88, Field memorandum no. 85-88. Geneva.

U.S. Committee for Refugees (1990). 1989 World refugee statistics. In *World Refugee Survey, 1989.* Washington, D.C.: American Council for Nationalities Service.

REFUGEE CHILDREN

I THEORETICAL OVERVIEWS

Refugee children present a complicated set of issues for those who wish to understand and assist them better. Premigration, transmigration, and postmigration experiences are frequently violent and traumatic. Adaptation to a new place and a new culture is another complicated process, during which the definition of family and of familial roles may change. This section reviews the mental health and sociological literatures as they pertain to refugee children.

In Chapter 1, Jean L. Athey and Frederick L. Ahearn identify and discuss the stressors commonly faced by refugee children. The more individualized stressors are outlined first, including trauma, loss, and deprivation, followed by an analysis of the ways in which the family may either buffer the effects of war, migration, and resettlement experiences or, on the other hand, add to the child's stress. Finally, the authors discuss how the refugee community and the larger society of which it is a part may affect the adjustment of child refugees.

John W. Berry discusses the meaning of "acculturation" for child refugees and their families in Chapter 2. He describes four ways in which adaptation—both the process and the outcome of dealing with acculturation—can be accomplished: assimilation, integration, separation, and marginalization. Variables specific to the host society, the refugee culture, and the individual effect which of these strategies dominate. Dr. Berry suggests that children may best be able to pursue the "integrationist" type of acculturation.

Neglect and abuse of refugee children after resettlement is a concern that is frequently raised. However, as discussed by Jill Korbin in Chapter 3, little is known about this subject. Dr. Korbin discusses the issues that need to be taken into account in any analysis of abuse, such as definitions and cultural practices that may be construed as abuse, and identifies avenues for future research.

1 The Mental Health of Refugee Children: An Overview

JEAN L. ATHEY, Ph.D., and
FREDERICK L. AHEARN, Jr., D.S.W.

Refugee experiences can range from the relatively benign, such as the migration of political or religious groups in intact families, to the horrific, including genocide, massive destruction, and the dissolution of community and family groups. Even the term *refugee* is open to dispute: sometimes it is used to mean anyone who flees from one country to another, and in other cases, particularly with governments, it distinguishes certain categories of legal from illegal entrants into a country. However, it most generally refers to persons who have fled from danger or oppression in one country or region and resettled in another. This volume focuses on children who not only have fled their countries of origin but also were exposed to considerable violence before or during their flights.

A comprehensive analysis of mental health issues for such children, the objective of this chapter, should take into account the many possibilities for personal, family, and community effects before, during, and after resettlement. The goal here is not to make a global assessment of how refugee children in general adjust to the numerous physical and psychological insults associated with their status, since there are so many variables that influence emotional well-being. Real-world categories of events, such as flight and migration, typically have multiple factors associated with them and they rarely have the quality of a laboratory control. For example, recent studies of the impact of divorce on children, a much more limited and well-defined experience than flight and resettlement in the context of violence, have shown that divorce varies tremendously along a number of dimensions, and thus, in order to understand its potential impact on a child, many different aspects of the divorce have to be characterized (Wallerstein and Corbin, 1989). This overview attempts to describe the possible variations in experiences for a refugee child and to identify the mental health and developmental

3

implications of such experiences and the potentiating or resilient factors children may bring to them.

However, children cannot be understood independently of their environments. Thus, an ecological framework is presented, with the child viewed as part of a family system and of a larger social system as well. The extent to which damage may ensue will in great part depend on the impact of violence and migration on the child's family and community.

Conceptually, this overview utilizes a stress model; it assumes that certain "stressors" require a child to "cope" and that the more powerful the stressor, the greater the resources needed by the child to cope successfully. The stress literature identifies numerous variables that are integrated into research models. These include genetic and other biological strengths and vulnerabilities, personality characteristics, particularly temperament and problem-solving skills, and the resources people can garner from various levels of the social system which help to protect them from negative effects of stress. However, the reactions of children, compared with adults, to stressful events remain an underresearched area.

Nevertheless, it is clear that certain events typically have negative consequences for children. Some may be so damaging that no child remains unscathed, although there may be variations in the form and severity of a child's reaction. In addition, children may be exposed to "sociocultural risk" in which the environment of the child is lacking in the basic social and psychological necessities for life. Thus, risk can be related either to direct threats or insults to the child or to impoverishment, the absence of opportunities for development (Garbarino, 1982). "At risk" or "developmental risk" is a statistical, epidemiological concept referring to increased risk of psychiatric morbidity, dysfunctional behavior patterns (such as suicide, drug and alcohol abuse, or delinquency), or "incompetence" in love, work, or play. However, "risk" is not destiny, and children can and do overcome adversity.

STRESS AND COPING FOR REFUGEE CHILDREN

The types of experience which many refugee children experience and which place a child at particular risk include trauma, loss, and severe deprivation. The coping behaviors that children employ when confronted with such stressors vary by developmental stage and by their ability to draw on various resources.

Trauma

Traumatic stressors have been defined as events perceived by the victim as a direct threat to life (either one's own or that of another) or as terrifying, horrifying, overwhelming, and outside the range of normal life experiences (Bolin, 1985). Eth and Pynoos (1985) defined a traumatic stressor as "an overwhelming event resulting in helplessness in the face of intolerable danger, anxiety, and instinctual arousal." In their view, trauma describes an intense experience involving all sensory modalities. Witnessing the infliction of injury, seeing a mutilated body, or coming near to death through violence are examples of traumatic stressors that may have profound impacts on adults as well as on children, sometimes leading to post-traumatic stress disorder (PTSD). Eth and Pynoos state that witnessing a relative's murder, a frequent experience of refugee children, always constitutes a psychic trauma.

Only a few studies have systematically examined trauma among children, and those that exist often have methodological problems or inadequate descriptions. Much of the literature on children in war situations, for example, does not distinguish among the types of event that the sampled children experienced. Some children living in war zones may not be exposed to traumatic stressors while others may have many such experiences, including witnessing the death or injury of a parent or sibling, or even continued and persistent exposure to death and destruction, as in Lebanon and Southeast Asia. Some children are tortured or are forced to witness torture (Allodi and Cowgill, 1982), while others are conscripted and forced to participate in violence.

One of the earliest and most often-cited war studies compared children who were sent out of London to avoid bomb attacks during World War II with a group who remained behind (Freud and Burlingham, 1943). The children who stayed with their parents in the city fared better than those who were sent to the country alone. The investigators concluded that separation from parents was more stressful than exposure to bombing. However, it is not clear whether the children who stayed actually experienced the bombing or whether they were personally confronted with death or destruction. The study identified the importance of the family as a buffer for stress and separation from the family as a major stressor, but it did not clearly address the impact of trauma on children.

More recent research has found severe and prolonged effects of traumatic events on children. A breakthrough study of traumatic stress in children was conducted by Newman (1976) with child victims of the dam break and flood at Buffalo Creek, West Virginia. Of 224 children interviewed, most were significantly impaired emotionally. Many had witnessed death and destruction and some had survived terrifying experiences. However, the study does not provide a clear picture of the effects of traumatic stress since these children were also deeply affected by the loss of their community. The study has also been criticized on methodological grounds, particularly with respect to sample selection.

Pynoos and Eth (1985) studied children who had witnessed the murder, rape, or suicide of a parent and found night terrors, startle reactions, intrusive imagery, and autonomous physiological reactions following these experiences. They reported that the reactions were the effects of the traumatic event and were different from those caused by the death of the parent. Physical injury of the child is identified as one important variable in the child's adjustment. Injured and uninjured children exposed to such trauma were found to have different reactions: the injured children were preoccupied with physical recovery and internal sensations and, unlike the uninjured children, were unable to deal immediately with the external trauma. They were found to be more prone to later dissociative symptoms, whereas this type of subsequent psychopathology was rare in uninjured child witnesses to violence.

Terr (1981) studied 26 children who had been kidnapped and buried alive in a bus in Chowchilla, California. Her study is particularly interesting since it involved children whose traumatic experience was not complicated by either bereavement or loss of community. Even 4 years after the event, these children had post-traumatic symptoms, including recurrent dreams of death, compulsive play, chronic anxiety, and personality changes. A more recent study of children traumatized by terrorism found that even 10 years later evidence of unresolved trauma remained (Dreman and Cohen, 1990).

These studies illustrate the severe effects that traumatic events can have on children. The way in which trauma is experienced and internalized is related to the age and developmental stage of the child. Preschoolers are particularly dependent on their parents and may react to trauma with anxious attachment behavior (Bowlby, 1980). School-age children often seem to adults to change radically following a traumatic event. They become irritable, rude, and argumentative or complain of somatic problems (Pynoos and Eth, 1984). School performance generally declines substantially. Adolescents are more like adults in their reactions. They may engage in antisocial acts or lose impulse control. They fear being ostracized because of the event, and they are frequently pessimistic about the future (Pynoos and Eth, 1984).

In sum, following exposure to a traumatic stressor, children experience symptoms of PTSD as well as cognitive and social deficits. The manifestations and severity of the reaction appear related to the degree of violence, presence or absence of personal injury, age of the child, and access to family support. However, as suggested in the limited number of studies of childhood trauma, such events rarely happen alone. This is particularly true for refugee children, who are also confronted with loss of family members or community.

Loss

Loss is a defining characteristic of refugee status. Children lose their homes, their possessions, their friends, and frequently their parents or siblings. For most children, the loss of a parent is an overwhelming disaster. Childhood bereavement can have major psychological ramifications, both immediate and long-term. Neurosis, depression, academic and social impairment, and delinquency have all been found to be intermediate outcomes of bereavement (Black, 1974; Raphael, 1983; Van Eerdewegh et al., 1982), while some studies have found adult mental illness to be related to childhood bereavement (Archibald et al., 1962; Barry, 1949). The developmental stage of the child at the time of parental or sibling death is particularly salient for the child's subsequent adjustment. The most vulnerable time appears to be the preschool years (Bowlby, 1980; Rutter, 1966) and early adolescence (Black, 1974).

A review of the literature on bereavement in children and adolescents identified 11 risk factors that increase the risk of psychological morbidity (Osterweis, Solomon, and Green, 1984). Whereas six of these may or may not apply to a given refugee child (e.g., age or gender), five of the risk factors are characteristic of the child refugee experience. Of these, two involve the mode of death: the risk of emotional problems is greater if the death is unanticipated or if the parent or sibling died through violence such as suicide or homicide. When a refugee child loses a parent, the death usually is unanticipated and involves violence.

Lack of adequate family or community supports is another risk factor for severe bereavement reactions; since the refugee child's experience typically consists of total disruption and even destruction of community, most are not able to access the supports that are so important for effective coping.

An unstable, inconsistent environment, including disruption of familiar routines, is a fourth risk factor common to refugee children. Rapidly changing environments with little stability for months or even years at a time is a common experience for a refugee child.

A fifth risk factor is the surviving parent's psychological vulnerability and excessive dependence on the child. Although psychological vulnerability has not been assessed in refugee parents, many have suffered greatly themselves and experience depression, anxiety, and other serious mental health problems. In short, the circumstances of parental and sibling death suggest that normal grieving and effective coping, which are difficult for any child who has lost a parent or sibling, are particularly problematic for most refugee children.

Refugee children also lose their homes. The sense of well-being, safety, and security for children is associated with familiarity of place, so loss of home can be extremely difficult, particularly if children do not feel protected by the adults in their lives (Coelho and Ahmed, 1980).

Deprivation

Severe deprivation in the form of insufficient food or water, lack of medical care, and inadequate housing is unfortunately characteristic of the lives of many of the world's children, both those who are living in or fleeing from zones of violence and those who are not. Refugee children frequently are severely deprived, sometimes for long periods, prior to or during migration or while in refugee camps. The physical health implications of deprivation may be more obvious than the mental health effects, but both occur; Carlin and Sokoloff (1985) report that Korean children malnourished because of the war demonstrated both physical and mental delays. Where physical development is stunted and survival questionable, cognitive and emotional impairments are likely. The degree of deprivation and how long it continues obviously affect the severity of the damage to a child's development.

Interaction Effects

While each type of experience—trauma, loss, and deprivation—has been discussed separately, they obviously happen to refugee children coterminously. Little research has been conducted on the interactive effects of such severe events on children; an exception is the work of Pynoos and Eth (1985), who found that the violence of a murder witnessed by a child generates "the trauma syndrome" (e.g., intrusive memories, startle reactions, nightmares, avoidant behavior) whereas the loss of a parent leads to "the grief syndrome" (e.g., sadness, anger, guilt, loneliness, preoccupation), and each places its own set of demands on a child. Pynoos and Eth suggest that children are particularly vulnerable "to the additive demands of trauma mastery and grief work." One complicates the other and makes each more difficult to successfully resolve.

Kinzie et al. (1986) examined a group of Cambodian refugee adolescents who had experienced severe trauma, loss, and deprivation and related their current functioning to their experiences prior to migration and to their current living situation. Four years after these traumatic experiences, half of the youths still experienced major symptoms of PTSD, such as nightmares, recurring dreams, being easily startled, and avoidance behavior. However, while the investigators did not find a simple relationship between reported experiences in Cambodia and psychiatric diagnosis—although they did find a strong relationship between the current living situation and psychiatric diagnosis—those youths who lived with a nuclear family member were much less likely to have a psychiatric problem than were those living in a foster family or living alone. This study documented the long-term effects of trauma, loss, and deprivation while highlighting the extreme importance of the family to the child's ability to withstand onslaughts and to work through even the most harrowing of experiences successfully.

Coping

The Kinzie et al. research could also be viewed as demonstrating coping outcomes. *Coping* has been defined as "behavior that protects the individual from internal and external stresses" (White, 1974). Alternatively, coping is viewed as "efforts both action-oriented and intrapsychic, to manage (i.e., master, tolerate, reduce, minimize) environmental and internal demands, and conflicts among them, which tax or exceed a person's resources" (Lazarus and Launier, 1978). People may engage in different forms of coping, such as changing the conditions that produce the stress; redefining the meaning of the stress experience as a way of de-emphasizing its significance; and manipulating the emotional consequences of the stress-producing experience so as to contain it within manageable bounds (Pearlin and Schooler, 1978). Children, as well as adults, may engage in these coping behaviors. Although coping incorporates behavioral responses, it also involves cognitive and perceptual processes. How particular events are defined and understood will greatly affect a refugee child's ability to, for example, avoid the source of stress, ignore a threat, or deny the outcome so as to maintain normal functioning.

Children who cope well with adverse situations have been referred to as "stress resistant" or "resilient" children. Both Rutter (1985) and Garmezy (1987) have studied those factors that help a child to overcome poor environments and stressful events. An important finding of Rutter's is that the more risk factors a child is exposed to, the more likely that he or she will have a psychiatric disorder. Thus, exposure to multiple stressors, both chronic and acute, greatly decreases a child's ability to cope successfully. As discussed above, refugee children typically confront many major stressors.

Garmezy (1987) identified three broad categories of variables that act as "protective factors" that assist a child in coping: (1) personality dispositions of the child, (2) a supportive milieu, and (3) an external support system that encourages and reinforces a child's coping efforts. When Garmezy examined stress outcomes in terms of "social competence" and "disruptiveness," he found that children with "greater assets" (higher IQ, higher socioeconomic status, and family stability and cohesion) fared better than those children with fewer such assets. "Social comprehension" was also important, a construct that included interpersonal understanding and problem-solving ability. Thus, these "assets" served as protective factors against stress. Werner's (1989) study of resilient children demonstrated that a very important characteristic of children who cope well with adverse circumstances is the ability to find emotional support in their community, either in addition to their immediate family or, when that family is unavailable or unsupportive, in place of the family.

Much remains to be learned about coping in children. The research on resilience in children and in particular on the relationship of developmental stage to coping is a fertile field for inquiry. However, it is already clear that the coping ability and style of children, including refugee children, is partly a function of their relationships with their parents, of their particular developmental levels, of personal temperament and intelligence, and of genetic factors all intertwined with their social resources. The quality of relationships with parents, siblings, significant relatives, neighbors, peers, and the larger society is also highly significant since it mediates these relationships (Rutter, 1983).

Bronfenbrenner (1979) suggests the importance of an ecological approach for analyzing the effects of changing and interdependent environmental forces on child development. His model examines the "person in environment" as a means to view the differential levels or contexts of human experience. This model is utilized in the following discussion of the refugee child within the family and neighborhood and the refugee child in the community. Bronfenbrenner's imperative to analyze environmental influences on development and on coping parallels the findings of Garmezy, Rutter, and Werner concerning the significance of family and other support systems if children are to cope effectively with major stressors.

THE REFUGEE FAMILY AND CHILD DEVELOPMENT

The family provides the basic security for a child which ensures that normal development can occur. Physical needs, protection from harm, and love are all provided by the family. The ability of the family to provide a strong sense of safety and support to the child and to serve as a buffer against external threats plays a large role in how well the child functions and develops. However, circumstances frequently impair the ability of refugee families from zones of violence to meet their children's needs adequately. For one thing, refugee families are frequently broken up or members lost, sometimes jeopardizing the child's physical survival or at least putting into question the ability of the remaining family members to provide for and protect the child. Depending on the age of the child, development can be seriously impaired by such family disruption.

Family disintegration can occur in several ways. Part or all of a child's family may be killed or accidentally separated from the child. In some cases, children are sent out of the country, sometimes with siblings and sometimes alone, while the parents remain. Alternatively, children may remain behind temporarily while part of the family leaves to get established in a new land, or they may be abducted into the army. Many months or even years may elapse by the time the child finally rejoins the family, and a whole new family may have been established. When the family is broken up in any of these ways, the level of safety and support available to the child is greatly diminished. Ressler, Boothby, and Steinbock (1988) point out that separation of a child from the mother is a major source of anxiety and developmental delay. Additional problems are created if the child must adjust to a new family configuration when families are reunited. Children placed in foster family situations typically have even greater problems (Kinzie et al., 1986).

Even if most of the family remains together, the adults may have difficulty in providing strong emotional support to children. Not infrequently the families of refugee children are suffering terrible stress and pain themselves and may therefore be unable to be adequately responsive to the child owing to their own stress and grief. Family members may be exposed to one or more traumatic events, even torture, and if so have their own serious reactions, such as PTSD. Parents, like their children, may experience grief over losses—loss of family members, of home, of valued possessions. Losses may also be psychological in nature, such as feelings of loss of safety, loss of status, or loss of control (Burgess and Holmstrom, 1984), or of violation of the self (Bard and Sangrey, 1979). These psychological losses may be particularly significant when violence is intentional and personally directed, as in torture or concentration camp experiences. Also, the sense of invulnerability, of basic safety and trust, may be lost, generating intense fear and anxiety (Perloff, 1983). If parents develop psychiatric morbidity, the illness can interfere with their ability to parent effectively. But even lower levels of stress can be detrimental to children; Freud and Burlingham (1943), for example, documented the significance of parental anxieties in provoking anxiety and stress symptoms in children.

In addition to anxiety, grief, and existential crises provoked by trauma and loss, refugee parents often experience radical changes in roles. If parents are separated, the remaining parent may have difficulty in fulfilling responsibilities that were once shared. The child may have lost a major source of nurturance and may also be expected to take on major adult responsibilities at a very early age. Furthermore, refugee parents are frequently dependent on a child for practical needs, particularly since the child may learn the new language of the settlement country much more quickly and easily than the parent. The child translates for the parent and often serves as the parent's cultural interpreter as well. Not infrequently, this situation becomes one of "status inconsistency" for the child—a situation in which a person occupies two or more distinct social statuses with incompatible social expectations leading to chronic stress (Canino, Earley, and Rogler, 1980). In short, the parents' grieving, anxiety reactions, and possible structural adjustments following loss of members may make it exceedingly difficult for parents to be as available and supportive to their children as they might otherwise be and as the child may need for optimum development.

The parents' ability to provide a sense of security, safety, and support to a child partly depends on a number of other factors: previous functioning of the family, the type of migration experience, and the social and economic resources of the family prior to and subsequent to becoming refugees, among others. Families that had serious problems before may find unresolved problems exacerbated; or the problems may be put on hold, so to speak, until the immediate crises are over but resurface upon resettlement. An example of this is family violence. Although the level of family violence, either spouse abuse or child abuse, has not been systematically studied among refugee families, it does sometimes occur. Family violence would be congruent with the literature on other populations in which violence frequently begets violence, with the victim becoming the perpetrator. When such violence occurs in a refugee child's family, the potential for greatly impaired functioning and developmental delays in the child is surely enhanced significantly. If, however, a family normally functions well, has adequate resources, and is able to stay together as a unit, it can greatly buffer the effects of stressors experienced by the child (Tsoi, Yu, and Lieh-Mak, 1986) and provide a safe enough environment for normal development to occur.

Even where family structures are weakened or members lost, children can often compensate for these deficiencies through their links with other systems such as school or church. The stronger these links, the more likely that the child's development will be positively influenced (Garbarino, 1982). A sense of personal competence improves a child's ability to forge such links. However, refugee children frequently have experiences that are potentially damaging to self-esteem and competence. For example, in school, whether in a refugee camp or in the settlement country, children are generally confronted with a new language and tend to fall behind academically. Identity problems can exacerbate school difficulties. Lack of success in school may become a major barrier to a sense of self-efficacy and to a child's ability to secure positive experiences outside the family. In short, refugee children may face formidable obstacles in securing affirming and strong linkages in the community.

THE LARGER COMMUNITY AND THE REFUGEE CHILD

Although *community* is often thought of as geography or place, it is best understood as the collective interests, values, and norms that organize activities and interactions. Community, in this sense, greatly influences self-identification and personal development as well as defining the relationships between oneself and others. Thus, it is not surprising that community disintegration has been linked with individual dysfunction in a number of studies. For example, Leighton's (1959) study of Nova Scotia demonstrated how economic breakdown, cultural confusion, and fragmented social supports led to interpersonal hostility, high rates of crime, and poor communication.

The destruction of a community's inner fabric or infrastructure has also been referred to as a "loss of community" (Erikson, 1976). Studying disaster victims in Buffalo Creek who had been dislocated, Erikson found that when individuals and families lost their connectedness with their locale, they also lost the support of people and institutions. The result, in many cases, was fear, insecurity, anger, anxiety, and depression. Refugee children and their parents typically experience disintegration of their original community, formation of a "flight community" (e.g., in a refugee camp) that may also subsequently break apart, and settlement in a totally new community. Two key aspects of community in understanding the impact of such change on children are culture and social relations.

Culture

Culture consists of the institutions, patterns, and mental attitudes that form the social life of the community (Sanders, 1966). In a sense, it is a collective understanding of what is, as well as the norms about what ought to be. Community as a collection of interests is mediated by culture. Culture becomes the glue that provides a community with meaning, cohesion, and integration.

Patterns and structures of socialization are the vehicles for passing on culture from generation to generation. Parents, schools, and religion are critical to this process. Refugee flight and resettlement, as discussed above, disrupt family life, often resulting in the inability of parents to socialize their children adequately. In addition, a major discontinuity of values and behavior patterns typically exists between the community of origin and that of settlement, including the prescribed and expected roles of individuals in the family. Traditional values may be called into question or made inappropriate by the pressures and reality of the new environment. Moreover, the functioning of the refugee family is disrupted as each member attempts differentially to adjust to the values of the new culture (Canino, Earley, and Rogler, 1980). One result of this pressure is an undermining of parental authority in general. Children more easily adapt to the new culture, assuming values that may clash with the expectations of traditional norms and generate intense familial conflict.

Schools also play a role in the socialization process. Both the form and content of schooling normally instill cultural identity and reinforce the standards of conduct and behavior learned at home. Refugee flight almost always disrupts this process in two ways: first, it breaks the continuity of the socialization process, and second, it prevents the child from progressing normally in learning information and skills. When the child reenters school in the settlement country, the socialization process continues, but it is socialization to a different culture. This schooling is typically discontinuous with the past and incongruent with the home environment.

Religion is the third major force in the socialization of the child, particularly in the inculcation of moral values to guide behavior. Religious values provide a framework for defining and dealing with problems. However, religious beliefs for child refugees from zones of violence have various ramifications. For some, faith and belief in a higher power may provide strength and support. Others, however, may lose their faith or angrily reject their religious heritage in the face of the atrocities they have witnessed. If the settlement country has a different religion, at a minimum the bonds to the old faith will usually be weakened as the child adjusts to the new environment.

In effect, then, many refugee children lose their strong cultural identities. Eisenbruck (1988) noted the significance of loss of culture when he discussed "cultural bereavement." He suggested that, in children, loss of culture leads to serious identity problems and delayed development. It is certainly a major task for a child to incorporate and superimpose what is meaningful and functional from one culture to another.

Social Relations

Communities are organized socially to provide security against common apprehensions. They provide a means of managing social relations, gaining associates, and establishing mutual intentions. The reestablishment of community in the settlement country may be problematic for several reasons.

First, the refugee family has experienced not only the inability of the community of origin to provide security but, in many cases, personal attacks by representatives of that community or of the larger society. Some refugees may have been so disillusioned by this betrayal that they become wary and suspicious of forming new community bonds. Second, and perhaps more significant, refugees are generally unversed in the dominant culture of the new society, may not know the language, and probably have difficulty interpreting nonverbal cues, thus making almost impossible the forms of mutual sharing that build trust and on which community is based. And third, political, ethnic, and racial antagonisms frequently impede the formation of a stable community.

Refugees face both within-group schisms and larger societal divisions. The preexisting ethnic, religious, and political divisions of the society of origin are frequently reinstituted in refugee groupings formed in the new country. These dissensions can sometimes be of great import, for example, when spies report (or are suspected of reporting) to the homeland on refugee activities with potentially severe repercussions for family members who have not yet escaped. Racism in the settlement society is also often a serious impediment to reestablishing a trustful and ordered community life. It stigmatizes and further isolates refugees. Finally, the class and social status of the refugee family may change within the larger society (e.g., a high-level official who becomes a taxi driver), leading to changes in self-perceptions and complicating the social relations among members of refugee groups.

Refugees may solve the problem of the profound disruption in social relations occasioned by flight and resettlement by restricting social relations to the safest ones; families can withdraw to their households and see only close relatives or, if possible, small groups of people who emigrated from the same geographic area. But reconstructing such a small social system takes considerable time.

The significance for refugee children of having no roots and a limited number of safe relationships can be profound. As discussed above, particularly when families cannot adequately support a child's coping, the larger community can sometimes compensate. But finding natural, external support is problematic for those refugee children who either individually or through the family have not been integrated into a new society in a meaningful way.

Finally, it is important to emphasize that the growth and development of refugee children are also associated with community systems beyond the neighborhood where decisions are made and policies implemented that greatly affect their lives and those of their parents. Economic and political systems, over which individuals have little if any influence, largely determine the conditions of refugee life. Day-to-day economic security, personal safety, and personal freedom are typically dependent on these outside forces—in the country of origin, the refugee camp, and the settlement country. Decision-making in these larger systems is rarely designed to enhance the growth and development of children.

CONCLUSION

This review has presented the problems faced by refugee children, on the assumption that such an understanding is essential to the design of effective policies and programs to assist these children. Such policies can be conceived of on three levels—societal, community, and individual. Clearly, the ideal solution is primary prevention—to prevent torture, violence, and family and community destruction. This battle must be fought in the political arena. While one may be less than sanguine about total prevention, clearly avenues can be pursued that may prevent at least some of this violence. Most programs and services focus on secondary prevention, at the community or individual level, or on treatment.

This overview suggests that policy and program development should be designed explicitly to strengthen communities and assist refugees in rebuilding their own communities within the larger society. Ways to support families should also be developed since the family is so critical to the child's adjustment. Direct support to the child, sometimes through mental health services, should also be offered, but in a manner consistent with the child's culture and sensitive to the child's place within the family and community. Such services, in short, should be child-centered and designed to support and strengthen families, should be culturally sophisticated, and should address the refugee child's emotional and developmental needs.

Finally, there are a number of things we do not know which we need to know. In order to set appropriate policies and plan culturally sensitive services for refugee children, more knowledge concerning short- and long-term consequences of refugee migration and adaptation is essential. For instance, how long do early symptoms of traumatic stress such as fear, nightmares, flashbacks, withdrawal or aggressive behavior, and eating and sleeping problems continue? Under what conditions are these symptoms mitigated? How frequently do children who do not initially exhibit emotional and physical problems develop them later? What are the best ways to provide support to children? Researchers need to examine these questions and others with longitudinal studies and demonstration programs.

Scholars and researchers are beginning to seek answers to these questions with systematic and methodologically sound procedures. Their findings and conclusions are now being disseminated to those who serve refugee children. This book is an effort toward this goal. As a whole it demonstrates that while the courage and resilience of refugee children are often formidable and demonstrate the power of their spirit, and while policies and programs should explicitly build on these strengths, it is incumbent on us to recognize that even the strongest child can be overwhelmed when the stresses are too great and the supports unavailable. When refugee children receive adequate support, assistance, and nurturing, however, they can and do develop into loving and competent persons, productive and secure.

REFERENCES

Allodi, F., and Cowgill, G. (1982). Ethical and psychiatric aspects of torture: A Canadian study. *Canadian Journal of Psychiatry, 27*, 98–102.

Archibald, H., Bell, D., Miller, C., and Tuddenham, R. (1962). Bereavement in childhood and adult psychiatric disturbance. *Psychosomatic Medicine, 4*, 343–51.

Bard, M., and Sangrey, D. (1979). *The Crime Victim's Book*. New York: Basic Books.

Barry, H. (1949). Significance of maternal bereavement before the age of eight in psychiatric patients. *Archives of Neurology and Psychiatry, 62*, 630–637.

Black, D. (1974). What happens to bereaved children? *Proceedings of the Royal Society of Medicine, 69*, 842–844.

Bolin, R. (1985). Disaster characteristics and psychosocial impacts. In B. J. Sowder (ed.), *Disasters and Mental Health: Selected contemporary perspectives*. Washington, D.C.: U.S. Government Printing Office.

Bowlby, J. (1980). *Attachment and Loss*, Vol. 3, *Loss*. New York: Basic Books.

Bronfenbrenner, U. (1979). *The Ecology of Human Development: Experiments by nature and design*. Cambridge, Mass.: Harvard University Press.

Burgess, A. W., and Holmstrom, L. L. (1984). Coping behavior of the rape victim. *American Journal of Psychiatry, 133*, 302–5.

Canino, I. A., Earley, B. F., and Rogler, L. H. (1980). *The Puerto Rican Child in New York City: Stress and Mental Health* (Monograph No. 4). New York: Hispanic Research Center, Fordham University.

Carlin, J. E., and Sokoloff, B. Z. (1985). Mental health treatment issues for Southeast Asian refugee children. In T. K. Owan (ed.), *Southeast Asian Mental Health: Treatment, Prevention, Services, Training, and Research,* pp. 91–112. U.S. Department of Health and Human Services publication ADM 85-1399. Rockville, Md.: National Institute of Mental Health.

Coehlo, G. V., and Ahmed, P. I. (eds.). (1980). *Uprooting and Development: Dilemmas of coping with modernization.* New York: Plenum.

Dreman, S., and Cohen, E. (1990). Children of victims of terrorism revisited: Integrating individual and family treatment approaches. *American Journal of Orthopsychiatry, 60*(2), 204–209.

Eisenbruck, M. (1988). The mental health of refugee children and their cultural development. *International Migration Review, 22*(2), 282–300.

Erikson, K. (1976). Loss of communality at Buffalo Creek. *American Journal of Psychiatry, 133,* 302–305.

Eth, S., and Pynoos, R. S. (1985). Interaction of trauma and grief in childhood. In S. Eth and R. S. Pynoos (eds.), *Post-traumatic Stress Disorder in Children,* pp. 168–186. Washington, D.C.: American Psychiatric Press.

Freud, A., and Burlingham, D. T. (1943). *War and Children.* New York: Ernst Willard.

Garbarino, J. (1982). *Children and Families in the Social Environment.* New York: Aldine.

Garmezy, N. (1987). Stress, competence, and development: Continuities in the study of schizophrenic adults, children vulnerable to psychopathology, and the search for stress-resistant children. *American Journal of Orthopsychiatry, 57*(2), 159–174.

Kinzie, J. D., Sack, W. H., Angell, R. H., Manson, S., and Rath, B. (1986). The psychiatric effects of massive trauma on Cambodian children: I. The children. *Journal of the American Academy of Child Psychiatry, 25,* 370–376.

Lazarus, R. S., and Launier, R. (1978). Stress-related transactions between person and environment. In L. A. Pervin and M. Lewis (eds.), *Perspectives in Interactional Psychology,* pp. 287–327. New York: Plenum.

Leighton, A. H. (1959). *My Name is Legion.* New York: Basic Books.

Newman, C. J. (1976). Children of disaster: Clinical observations at Buffalo Creek. *American Journal of Psychiatry, 133,* 306–12.

Osterweis, M., Solomon, F., and Green, M. (eds.). (1984). *Bereavement, Reactions, Consequences, and Care.* Washington, D.C.: Institute of Medicine, National Academy of Sciences.

Pearlin, L. I., and Schooler, C. (1978). The structure of coping. *Journal of Health and Social Behavior, 19,* 548–555.

Perloff, L. S. (1983). Perceptions of vulnerability to victimization. *Journal of Social Issues, 39,* 41–62.

Pynoos, R. S., and Eth, S. (1984). The child as witness to homicide. *Journal of Social Issues, 40,* 87–108.

Pynoos, R. S., and Eth, S. (1985). Children traumatized by witnessing acts of personal violence: Homicide, rape, or suicide behavior. In S. Eth and R. S. Pynoos (eds.), *Post-traumatic Stress Disorder in Children*, pp. 17–43. Washington, D.C.: American Psychiatric Press.

Raphael, B. (1983). *The Anatomy of Bereavement.* New York: Basic Books.

Ressler, E. M., Boothby, N., and Steinbock, D. J. (1988). *Unaccompanied Children.* New York: Oxford University Press.

Rutter, M. (1966). *Children of Sick Parents.* London: Oxford University Press.

Rutter, M. (1983). Stress, coping, and development: Some issues and some questions. In N. Garmezy and M. Rutter (eds.), *Stress, Coping, and Development in Children*, pp. 1–41. New York: McGraw-Hill.

Rutter, M. (1985). Resilience in the face of adversity: Protective factors and resistance to psychiatric disorder. *British Journal of Psychiatry, 147,* 598–611.

Sanders, I. (1966). *Community: An Introduction to a Social System.* New York: Ronald Press.

Terr, L. C. (1981). Forbidden games. *Journal of the American Academy of Child Psychiatry, 20,* 741–760.

Tsoi, M. M., Yu, G. K. K., and Lieh-Mak, F. (1986). Vietnamese refugee children in camps in Hong Kong. *Social Science and Medicine, 23,* 1147–1150.

Van Eerdewegh, M., Bieri, M., Parilla, R., and Clayton, P. (1982). The bereaved child. *British Journal of Psychiatry, 140,* 23–29.

Wallerstein, J. S., and Corbin, S. B. (1989). Daughters of divorce: Report from a ten-year follow-up. *American Journal of Orthopsychiatry, 59*(4), 605–618.

Werner, E. E. (1989). High risk children in young adulthood: A longitudinal study from birth to 32 years. *American Journal of Orthopsychiatry, 59*(1), 72–81.

White, R. W. (1974). Strategies of adaptation: An attempt at systematic description. In G. V. Coehlo, D. A. Hamburg, and J. E. Adams (eds.), *Coping and Adaptation*, pp. 47–68. New York: Basic Books.

2 Refugee Adaptation in Settlement Countries: An Overview with an Emphasis on Primary Prevention

JOHN W. BERRY, Ph.D.

This chapter attempts to provide an overview, from the perspective of cross-cultural psychology, of the factors that may govern the relationship between acculturation and mental health in refugee populations. One fundamental assumption is that individuals *can* move successfully between cultures (even refugees who have been exposed to war and other traumatic experiences); another is that this process of acculturation can be *managed* (by individuals and agencies) to increase the probability of successful adaptation and to reduce or even prevent mental problems.

In preparing this overview, I have drawn on academic reviews of this issue (e.g., Berry, 1986; Berry and Kim, 1988; Canadian Task Force, 1986; Lam, 1987; Westermeyer, 1986; Williams, 1987); on empirical research programs (e.g., Beiser, 1986; Berry et al., 1987; Westermeyer, 1987); and on reports of recent consultations among refugee mental health personnel (e.g., League of Red Cross and Red Crescent Societies, 1986, 1987; Refugee Action, 1987).

My approach is to provide a general description of the processes of acculturation and adaptation and then to indicate what the general literature tells us about how individuals and groups can achieve a successful outcome. Then I turn specifically to the case of refugees, particularly refugee children (United Nations High Commission for Refugees, 1988), applying the general principles to their special situation.

It is obvious to all of us that a process of culture contact and change has been taking place for millennia and continues at an ever-increasing pace. In the past, conquest and enslavement were common, while nowadays migration (both voluntary and enforced) is the predominant experience. Individuals and groups must somehow deal with this process in all its dimensions: political, economic, cultural, social, and psychological. In this chapter, the concepts of acculturation and adaptation will be employed to describe and analyze the overall chain of events from

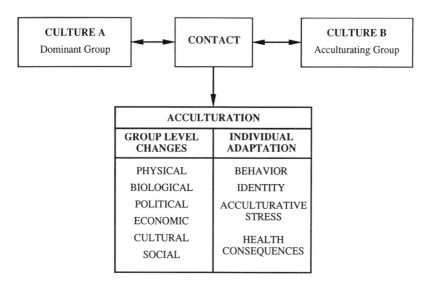

Figure 2.1. The process of acculturation and adaptation

initial contact to the eventual mental health consequences for the individual. While the analysis is cast in general terms (that is, for all acculturating peoples), the assumption is made that the psychological processes of adaptation are similar among refugees and asylum seekers and that we can better serve this special group by understanding the general phenomena of acculturation and psychological adaptation.

THEORETICAL PERSPECTIVES

Acculturation

Acculturation is a term that has been defined as a cultural exchange that results from continuous, first-hand contact between two distinct cultural groups (Redfield, Linton, and Herskovits, 1936) (Figure 2.1). While originally proposed as a group-level phenomenon, it is now also widely recognized as an individual-level phenomenon, and is termed *psychological acculturation* (Graves, 1967). At this second level, acculturation refers to changes in an individual (both overt behavior and covert traits) whose cultural group is collectively experiencing acculturation. It is important to note here that, while mutual changes are implied in the definition, in fact most changes occur in the nondominant group (culture B) as a result of influence from the dominant group (culture A). It is on these nondominant (or acculturating) groups that we will focus in trying to link acculturation experience to psychological adaptation.

What kinds of change may occur as a result of acculturation? First, physical changes: a new place to live, a new type of housing, increasing population density, urbanization, more pollution, etc., are all common with acculturation. Second, biological changes may occur; new nutritional status and new diseases (often devastating in force) are all common. Third, political changes may take place, usually bringing the nondominant groups under some degree of control, and usually involving some loss of autonomy. Fourth, economic changes may occur, which consist of people moving away from traditional pursuits toward new forms of employment. Fifth, cultural changes (which are at the heart of the definition) necessarily occur; original linguistic, religious, educational, and technical institutions become altered or imported ones take their place. Sixth, social relationships, including intergroup and interpersonal relations, become altered, and new patterns of dominance may appear. Finally, numerous psychological changes may appear at the individual level. Changes in behavior are well documented in the literature (see Berry, 1980, for a review); these include, for example, changes in values, abilities, and motives. Existing identities and attitudes change and new ones develop: self-attitudes (personal identity and ethnic identity) often shift away from those held prior to contact, and views about how (and whether) one should participate in the process of acculturation emerge (Berry et al., 1989). Other attitudes (such as intergroup attitudes and lifestyle preferences) also change and develop during acculturation.

Stress phenomena and related pathology both appear during acculturation (Berry et al., 1987). Although these negative and largely unwanted consequences of acculturation are not inevitable, and although there are also opportunities to be encountered during acculturation, it is nevertheless true that serious problems do appear in relation to acculturation (Berry and Kim, 1988). These problems reside in the interaction between the two groups in contact, and they can be managed and ameliorated by identifying their specific source and by restructuring the relationships between the groups.

Adaptation

As employed here, *adaptation* is the generic term used to refer to both the process of dealing with acculturation and the outcome of acculturation. At the outset, we need to recognize that the concept of adaptation has a long and complex history in the social and behavioral sciences: psychologists can study how individuals come to grips with the social, cultural, or ecological setting in which they find themselves (Honig-mann, 1976).

In all disciplines, though, it is accepted that there are different strategies of adaptation (as a process) which lead to different varieties of adaptation (as an outcome). For the individual, three such strategies have been identified (Berry, 1976). These have been termed *adjustment, reaction,* and *withdrawal,* and they may be identified in the following way. With adjustment, changes in the organism are in a direction that reduces the conflict (i.e., increases the congruence or fit) between the environment and the organism by bringing it into harmony with the environment. In general, this strategy is the one most often intended by the term *adaptation* and may indeed be the commonest form. With reaction, changes are in a direction that retaliates against the environment; these may lead to environmental changes that, in effect, increase the congruence or fit between the two, but not by way of cultural or behavioral adjustment. In the case of withdrawal, change is in a direction that reduces the pressures from the environment; in a sense, it is a removal from the adaptive arena and can occur either by forced exclusion or by voluntary withdrawal.

It is important to note that the third strategy, withdrawal, is often not a real possibility for those being influenced by larger and more powerful cultural systems. And for the second strategy, reaction, in the absence of political power to divert acculturative pressures, many acculturating peoples cannot successfully engage in retaliatory responses. Thus, individual change in order to adapt to the context (some form of the adjustment strategy of adaptation) is often the only realistic alternative.

Just as there are strategies of adaptation, so too there are varying ways in which individuals can acculturate. Corresponding to the view that adjustment is not the only strategy of adaptation, I take the view that assimilation is not the only mode of acculturation. This position becomes clear when we examine the framework proposed by Berry (1984) (Figure 2.2). The model is based on the observation that in culturally plural societies, individuals and groups must confront two important issues. One pertains to the maintenance and development of one's ethnic distinctiveness in society; it must be decided whether one's own cultural identity and customs are of value and should be retained. The other issue involves the desirability of interethnic contact, deciding whether relations with the larger society are of value and should be sought. These are essentially questions of attitudes and values and may be responded to on a continuous scale, from positive to negative. For conceptual purposes, however, they can be treated as dichotomous (yes or no) decisions, thus generating a fourfold model (see Figure 2.2) that

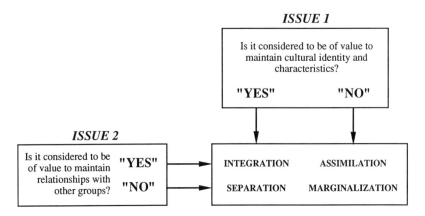

Figure 2.2. Four modes of acculturation

serves as the basis for our discussion. Each cell in this fourfold classification is considered to be an acculturation option (both a strategy and an outcome) available to individuals and to groups in plural societies. These four options are *assimilation, integration, separation,* and *marginalization.*

The *assimilation* option is defined as relinquishing one's cultural identity and moving into the larger society. It can take place by absorbing a nondominant group into an established dominant group by merging many groups to form a new society, as in the "melting pot" concept. This is clearly the variety that most closely resembles the adjustment form of adaptation.

The *integration* option implies some maintenance of the cultural integrity of the group (i.e., some reaction to acculturative pressures) as well as the movement to become an integral part of a larger societal framework (i.e., some adjustment). Therefore, in the case of integration, the option taken is to retain cultural identity and move to join with the dominant society. In this case, there are a number of distinguishable ethnic groups, all cooperating within a larger social system.

When no substantial relations with the larger society is accompanied by a maintenance of ethnic identity and traditions another option is defined. Depending upon which group (the dominant or nondominant) controls the situation, this option may take the form either of segregation or of *separation.* When the pattern is imposed by the dominant group, segregation to keep people in "their place" appears (i.e., reaction followed by exclusion). On the other hand, the maintenance of a traditional way of life outside full participation in the larger society may be desired by the acculturating group and thus lead to an independent existence, as in the case of separatist movements (i.e., reaction followed by withdrawal). In our terms, segregation and separation differ mainly with respect to which group or groups have the power to determine the outcome.

Finally, there is an option that is difficult to define precisely, possibly because it is accompanied by a good deal of collective and individual confusion and stress. It is characterized by striking out against the larger society and by feelings of alienation, loss of identity, and what has been termed acculturative stress (Berry and Annis, 1974). This option is *marginalization*, in which groups lose cultural and psychological contact with their traditional culture and the larger society (either by exclusion or withdrawal). When imposed by the larger society, it is tantamount to ethnocide. When stabilized in a nondominant group, it constitutes the classic situation of marginality (Stonequist, 1937).

Two points should be made with respect to the model in Figure 2.2. First, the various options may be pursued by politically dominant or nondominant groups. Second, the model in Figure 2.2 can be employed at three distinct levels. First, at the level of the dominant or larger society, national policies can be identified as those encouraging assimilation, integration, separation and segregation, or marginalization. For example, in Canada the official policy is clearly one of integration (termed *multiculturalism* by the federal government), whereas other societies' policies can be identified as inclining toward other alternatives, using this framework. Second, at the level of acculturating groups, these communities can articulate their wishes and goals and communicate them to their members and to the larger society. Third, at the level of individuals, attitudes toward these four alternatives can be assessed using standard attitude measurement techniques to obtain individual preferences about which mode of acculturation is most desirable (see Berry et al., 1986, for a review of some empirical studies of acculturation attitudes).

RESEARCH FINDINGS

Acculturating Groups

Although many of the generalities found in the literature about the effects of acculturation have been based on a single type of group, it is clear that there are numerous types, and adaptations may vary depending upon this factor.

In the review by Berry and Kim (1988), five different groups were identified: immigrants, refugees, native peoples, ethnic groups, and sojourners (Figure 2.3). There are variations in the degree of voluntariness,

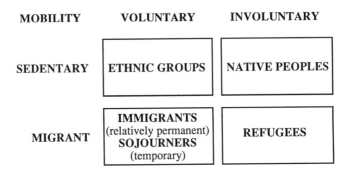

Figure 2.3. Five types of acculturating groups

movement, and permanence of contact, all factors that might affect the health of members of the group. Those who are voluntarily involved in the acculturation process (e.g., immigrants) may experience less difficulty than those with little choice in the matter (e.g., refugees and native peoples), since their initial attitudes toward contact and change may be more positive. Further, those only temporarily in contact and who are without permanent social supports (e.g., sojourners) may experience more health problems than those more permanently settled and established (e.g., ethnic groups). These distinctions suggest some important variations in outcomes which are subject to empirical verifications during the course of the research.

Dominant Groups

Variations in dominant groups also exist, and these variations may have implications for the health of acculturating people. First, there are clear variations in the degree to which the maintenance of cultural diversity is tolerated. As Murphy (1965) noted, tolerant (pluralist, multicultural) societies do not generally force individuals to change their ways of life, and they usually have viable ethnic social support groups to assist individuals in the acculturation process. In contrast, monistic societies place more pressures on acculturating individuals to change, and often lack social supports for them. Both of these factors have clear implications for the social and mental health of acculturating individuals.

Second, even in relatively pluralistic and tolerant societies, all ethnic groups are not equally accepted; variations in ethnic attitudes in the larger society (including levels of prejudice and acts of discrimination) are well documented for Canada (Berry, Kalin, and Taylor, 1977) and for many other countries.

Acculturative Stress

The concept of stress has had wide usage in the psychological and medical literature (Selye, 1975, 1976), and it has sparked considerable controversy as well. There is no intention here to present a formal definition or conceptual model of stress. For the purposes of this chapter, *stress* is considered to be a generalized physiological and psychological state of the organism, which is brought about by the experience of stressors in the environment and which requires some reduction (for normal functioning to occur), through a process of coping, until some satisfactory adaptation to the new situation is achieved.

The concept of acculturative stress refers to one kind of stress, in which the stressors are identified as having their source in the process of acculturation; in addition, there is often a particular set of stress behaviors that occur during acculturation, such as lowered mental health status (specifically, confusion, anxiety, depression), feelings of marginality and alienation, heightened psychosomatic symptom level, and confused identity. Acculturative stress is thus a phenomenon that may underlie poor health in individuals (including physical, psychological, and social aspects). To qualify as acculturative stress, these changes should be related in a systematic way to known features of the acculturation process, as experienced by the individual.

In a recent review and integration of the literature, Berry and Kim (1988) attempted to identify the cultural and psychological factors that govern the relationship between acculturation and mental health. We concluded that, clearly, mental health problems often do arise during acculturation; however, these problems are not inevitable and seem to depend on a variety of group and individual characteristics that enter into the acculturation process. That is, acculturation sometimes enhances one's life chances and mental health and sometimes virtually destroys one's ability to carry on; the eventual outcome for any particular individual is affected by other variables that govern the relationship between acculturation and stress.

This conception is illustrated in Figure 2.4. On the left of the figure, acculturation occurs in a particular situation (e.g., migrant community or native settlement) and individuals participate in and experience these changes to varying degrees; thus, individual acculturation experience may vary from a great deal to rather little. In the middle, stressors may result from this varying experience of acculturation; for some people, acculturative changes may all be in the form of stressors, while for oth-

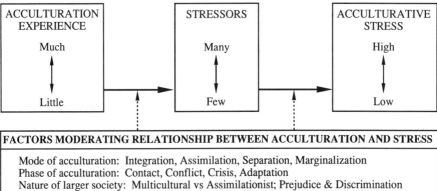

Figure 2.4. Factors relevant to acculturative stress

ers, they may be benign or even seen as opportunities. On the right, varying levels of acculturative stress may become manifest as a result of acculturation experience and stressors.

The first crucial point to note is that relationships among these three concepts (indicated by the solid horizontal arrows) are probabalistic, rather than deterministic; the relationships are likely to occur, but are not fixed. The second crucial point is that these relationships all depend on a number of moderating factors (indicated in the lower box), including the nature of the larger society, the type of acculturating group, the mode of acculturation being experienced, and a number of demographic, social, and psychological characteristics (including coping abilities) of the group and individual members. That is, each of these factors can influence the degree and direction of the relationships between the three variables at the top of Figure 2.4. This influence is indicated by the broken vertical arrows drawn between this set of moderating factors and the horizontal arrows.

One of these moderating factors, as we have already seen, is the nature of the host or larger society. Is there a pluralist or multicultural ideology (with attendant tolerance for cultural diversity), or is there an assimilationist ideology (with pressures to conform to a single cultural standard)? As we have noted, arguments, and some evidence, exist (e.g., Murphy, 1965) that health problems may be less among immigrants in plural societies than in assimilationist ones.

Other variables identified by Berry and Kim (1988) were the nature of the acculturating group (immigrants, refugees, native peoples, ethnic groups, and sojourners), modes of acculturation (assimilation, integration, separation and segregation, and marginalization), and a variety of demographic, social, and psychological characteristics of the individual. These are generally in the domain of "psychosocial factors" (World Health Organization, 1979) and include characteristics such as premigration experiences (war, torture, or famine), prior cultural knowledge and encounters (essentially a form of "preacculturation"), age, gender, marital status, social supports, a sense of "cognitive control" that one has over the acculturation process, and the degree of congruity between one's expectations about the acculturation process and the realities one has encountered during the process. Of particular importance among these psychological factors is the individual's ability to cope with acculturative experience; individuals are known to vary widely in how they deal with major changes in their lives (Lazarus and Folkman, 1984), resulting in large variations in the levels of stress experienced. Many other factors appear in the literature, but in our review these seemed to be the most theoretically relevant, and empirically consistent, predictors of acculturative stress.

PHASES OF ACCULTURATION

Experiences that are related to psychological acculturation and eventual adaptation may be classified sensibly according to the time (or phase) at which they take place. Such a classification should not be taken to imply that there is a standard experience or that it takes place at a standard pace or within a set period of time. For refugees, these phases may be termed predeparture, flight, first asylum, claimant period, settlement period, and adaptation. In each phase there are some experiences that are unique (e.g., torture) and some that are common with other phases (e.g., uncertainty). In this section I attempt to identify these characteristic experiences, to place them in a generalized time frame (Figure 2.5), and to consider their potential implications for prevention of psychological and social problems.

Predeparture

In the predeparture period there exist the most traumatic events that put refugees at risk for later development of mental and social problems. Ironically, it is these very high risk factors that are least amenable to prevention by those in the mental health field. However, international and civil wars, revolutions, famines, and ecological disasters are not "natural" events; they are the result of human action and are thus amenable to human counteraction. The largest refugee dislocations at the

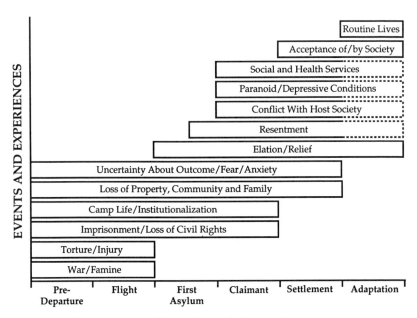

Figure 2.5. Phases, events, and experiences during a refugee career

present time are those due to military interventions (either direct or indirect) by major world powers and to the long and painful process of decolonization. A fundamental program in primary prevention, then, would address these macroproblems on an international scale; and we in refugee-receiving countries are in a position to bring about some amelioration.

Within nation states, other more direct factors are evident: ethnic, racial, and religious conflict and persecution, political violence, imprisonment, and deliberate torture (Barudy, 1987; Horvath, 1987) all become compounded in the accumulation of predeparture trauma. These situations, too, are the result of human actions and in principle are subject to human counteraction. Primary prevention is thus not beyond contemplation; however, we in receiving nations may be less capable of improving these largely internal situations.

In short, fundamentally important events in the experience of trauma are least within our primary prevention purview as mental health professionals, but they can be addressed in public from our professional platforms. Common sense suggests that we should be addressing these big and difficult issues at the same time as we attempt to deal with the relatively small but more accessible ones. Making daily repairs to continually breaking parts of a faulty machine is of limited long-term usefulness.

Flight

During flight the trauma usually continues, with the same attendant risks of capture (or recapture), privation, starvation, and of physical injury, even death. Loss of property, community, and family and uncertainty about what awaits one at the end of the journey have direct psychological impact. Once again, no primary prevention is possible during flight, but improving knowledge of the usual experiences during this phase on the part of mental health professionals should enhance the usefulness of later primary prevention.

First Asylum

Immediate elation and relief are often experienced on arrival in first asylum situations. In border areas especially, however, continuing fear for personal safety continues, as well as uncertainty. For most refugees, some sort of camp, even imprisonment, also continues. Although first asylum is, in principle, available to all who physically arrive, both at this phase and at the next point (claimant phase) the refugee is subject to deportation either to his or her country of origin or to another country of first asylum. On the recognition that most of one's problems are likely to continue for many years, elation and relief may give way to resentment and to a resurgence of uncertainty, fear, and anxiety; this has been termed "delayed psychology entry" by Tyhurst (1980).

During camp or community life in the phase of first asylum, some primary prevention is possible (Fozzard, 1987). However, safety and physical needs are usually paramount, and psychological needs may go unexpressed, unidentified, or unmet. Retrospective accounts by refugees and previous experiences of camp-working professionals can provide much needed information for the development of primary mental health programs at this phase.

In their highly informative document on refugee children, the United Nations High Commission for Refugees (1988) has pointed out how much positive activity can be accomplished for children during the first asylum phase. Particularly in organized camps, the protection of children and the meeting of their physical, social, and psychological health needs can be pursued quickly and efficiently given appropriate camp resources and organization. Often, too, there are resources for children within the refugee population: many adults will have parenting skills, and perhaps professional or paraprofessional training in working with children. Programs to promote infant stimulation and play and social integration of children in peer and adult groups can be successfully pursued with such internal resources. In cases of family separation (resulting in the presence of "unaccompanied minors"), early efforts at family tracing and reunification should be made. For such children, care can be provided by members of their own community (regional, religious, or ethnic); this community involvement assists in cultural maintenance and the development of a sense of belonging. For longer-term programs, nonformal and formal (primary and secondary) education can be provided, sometimes as part of the host national educational system and sometimes using resources in the refugee population, in efforts to develop literacy and numeracy skills.

Claimant

Once again, in principle, all claimants for refugee status are entitled to be granted asylum by countries who have signed the United Nations convention. In practice, however, many are turned away, and knowledge of this possibility can raise uncertainty and fear to unbearable levels. If deportation is ordered, the claimant is often left entirely without support, and suicide is not uncommon. If asylum is granted, elation and relief continue, often followed by resentment at being in limbo between flight and settlement. Conflict with officials and sometimes hostile citizens of the host society also frequently develops. Depending on the host country, there is large variation in work rules, educational possibilities, and the availability of health and social services during this phase. In one formulation, this is a severely marginalized situation, in which very high levels of acculturative stress can begin to appear (as distinct from the stress of flight). In extreme cases, paranoid conditions and depression become common during this phase.

Primary prevention may be particularly effective here; however, social and health care may be unavailable or be in dispute among authorities. Even effectively functioning or professionally trained individuals within the refugee community may be prevented from acting on behalf of fellow refugees, in some countries. Despite these impediments, the claimant period offers the most available time period for prevention work. For it is in this period that a set of necessary preconditions exists: relative safety, met physical needs, some degree of settled life, usable time, and (potentially) available services. Refugee-receiving countries may be able to make best use of their humanitarian resources during this phase, even if all claimants will not eventually be admitted.

Settlement

By far most primary prevention is possible here, for at this point the host society formally accepts the refugee as a potential citizen, usually with all the rights and freedoms granted to citizens. Unfortunately, as pointed out by many observers (e.g., Westermeyer, 1987; Williams, 1987), many settlement programs have not taken advice from mental health professionals, have not learned from previous refugee waves, and have not been formally evaluated. In some cases settlement policies have been clearly inappropriate: scattering or dispersal of families or communities during settlement wipes out needed social support and induces assimilation; sponsors have sometimes sought cheap labor or converts; health and social services are frequently culturally inappropriate; service providers are culturally ignorant or insensitive; and services may be much too short-lived to be of value.

For children, attempts should be made to maintain their relationships with other family members or, if this is not possible, with those who share their language, culture, and identity. Such social support systems are now known to be extremely important for all persons experiencing acculturation; they can be no less so for the developing child. In particular, well-meaning attempts to "provide the best" for refugee children can really impose unnecessary assimilative pressures on vulnerable children, leading to identity loss and a sense of marginalization.

Despite these problems, reports from Western Europe, Canada, and the United States indicate that most refugees settle without serious difficulty, given basic minimal services of language training, initial social and monetary support, and cultural orientation to the new society; that is, there is a gradual acceptance of, and by, the host society. Those with particularly traumatic histories, however, still need to be identified early and validly, using culturally appropriate instruments, and culturally sensitive personnel. Thus, during the settlement phase the needs are twofold: basic preventive services for the whole refugee population (including screening) and specialized services for those at particular risk.

Adaptation

While not all refugees adapt satisfactorily to their new society, most eventually do, and settle into routine lives. Evidence from earlier waves of migrants from Europe and elsewhere (e.g., Hungary, Uganda, Chile, Cuba) suggests that the long-term prognosis is rather good. However, comparisons and generalizations like this ignore variations in many of the factors identified in Figure 2.4, and caution is necessary. One source of caution is particularly relevant: in the past few years elderly refugees from earlier waves have begun to ask for treatment in mental health services, suggesting that a stable adaptation may be only a temporary achievement (Rack, 1987).

In contrast, children, because they are more adaptable (particularly with respect to language and the acquisition of social skills), may have an especially good potential for pursuing the integrative mode of acculturation; this, of course, requires reasonable access to both heritage and host cultures, and a freedom of choice to live with both cultural traditions. However, the risk of marginalization is particularly high during adolescence, and special care must be taken to give adolescents access to both cultures, so that they do not develop the feeling of being trapped in limbo, between cultures.

IMPLICATIONS AND CONCLUSIONS

The factors associated with the mental health of refugees in this overview are just that—"associated." We have relied upon correlational and observational data; in the virtual absence of longitudinal and evaluative studies and the complete absence of experimental studies that may link cause and effect together in a more formal way, we can take as only hints or suggestions that certain conditions may lead to certain outcomes. As replications build up and as comparative studies permit the teasing out of specific factors one from another, we may claim more and more validity; but the field of refugee mental health is inherently incapable of experimental attack. Thus, it is necessary to keep these limitations in mind when asserting some basis for policy action.

With these cautions in mind, we may make a number of observations and assertions. First, viewed in the light of these general principles and processes of acculturation and psychological adaptation, refugees and asylum seekers are clearly more at risk than other groups of acculturating peoples. This position needs to be firmly established and the evidence clearly understood if remedial action, in terms of policies and programs, is to be developed, accepted, and implemented.

Reviewing the general framework that has been presented, with a specific focus on refugees, we note the following.

Figure 2.1

Dominant groups are often very dominant with respect to a relatively powerless group of refugees; this imbalance in demographic, military, political, and economic power is likely to produce an extremely difficult situation for the refugees. In turn, group-level changes, including physical conditions (housing and safety), malnutrition and sanitary conditions, political isolation, economic loss, and cultural and social disintegration are likely to be much worse for refugees than for any other type of acculturating group. Individual adaptations are consequently also likely to be extreme, with major changes in daily behavior (due to loss of independence, in sometimes prisonlike conditions), loss of identity and confusion, and the probability of intense levels of stress. Consequences for health, but in particular mental health problems, are thus most likely to be extreme for refugees and asylum seekers.

Figure 2.2

Countries of first asylum may be those that are least able, politically or economically, to permit full participation of the new arrivals; hence the assimilation and integration modes of acculturation are less likely to occur than the segregation or marginalization options. This reality places certain limitations on the choices that refugees themselves can make, and any discrepancy between one's own preferences and those permitted by the host society are likely to create stressors for the refugees.

Figure 2.3

The research literature has clearly shown that two factors, voluntariness and mobility, are important in stress induction. It is obvious that refugees are getting the worst from both of these conditions, leading to the expectation that stress will be greater for them than for any other kind of acculturating group. Lacking positive motivation ("pull factors") to move—and with an abundance of "push factors"—and being unable to maintain a supportive political, economic, and sociocultural context, refugees are forced to exist in the worst of all acculturating worlds. Moreover, like sojourners, asylum seekers must live with a temporary and uncertain status, leading to extra stressors.

Figure 2.4

At the crux of the analysis is the probabalistic sequence: acculturation experiences—stressors—acculturative stress (moderated by numerous contextual and psychological factors). Without enumerating once again those variables identified in Figures 2.1 through 2.3, it is clear that almost all of the probabalistic factors in Figure 2.4 are weighted against a positive adaptation for refugees and asylum seekers.

Figure 2.5

The time course of being a refugee clearly places the major stressors at the beginning, with the *possibility* of improvement later. Countries of first asylum and the eventual countries of settlement can choose to either assist in this improvement, or they can perpetuate the trauma by bringing new stressors to bear on the refugee. It appears that refugee policies and programs may have come closer to the latter alternative, whether intended or not.

Despite this rather negative observation, most of the factors identified here are under some degree of control by those responsible for creating a refugee situation in the first place, by those serving as countries of first asylum, by those serving as resettlement countries, and by the refugees themselves. Each of these points of entry into the problems can serve as a point of partial control over the sequence. Armed with a knowledge of the acculturation process, and of the critical variables involved, efforts can be made to alter the probabilities toward more positive adaptations. It is, of course, a monumental task, but it is a possible one.

It is important to note that no psychological finding (or theory or method) can be transported or generalized to other cultures. Thus, the present overview is intended to stimulate and to challenge research on psychological acculturation and refugee adaptation, rather than to be taken uncritically as the proper way to do things or as a statement of the inevitable outcomes of acculturation. Variations, due to factors in the host society and in the acculturating group and to individuals involved in the process, will all make the results highly variable from one society, group, and person to another. Perhaps it is this emphasis on individual and group variability that psychologists have the most to contribute to the study of refugees and asylum seekers.

REFERENCES

Barudy, J. (1987). *Psychotherapy among Latin American torture victims in Belgium.* Paper presented at Workshop on Refugee Children's Mental Health. Refugee Studies Centre, Oxford University.

Beiser, M. (1986). Measuring psychiatric disorder among Southeast Asian refugees. *Psychological Medicine, 16,* 627–639.

Berry, J. W. (1976). *Human Ecology and Cognitive Style: Comparative Studies in Cultural and Psychological Adaptation.* London: Sage.

Berry, J. W. (1980). Social and cultural change. In H. C. Triandis and R. Brislin (eds.), *Handbook of Cross-Cultural Psychology,* Vol. 5, *Social,* pp. 211–279. Boston: Allyn & Bacon.

Berry, J. W. (1984). Cultural relations in plural societies: Alternatives to segregation and their sociopsychological implications. In N. Miller and M. Brewer (eds.), *Groups in Contact*, pp. 11–27. New York: Academic Press.

Berry, J. W. (1986). The acculturation process and refugee behavior. In C. L. Williams and J. Westermeyer (eds.), *Refugee Mental Health in Resettlement Countries*, pp. 25–37. Washington, D.C.: Hemisphere.

Berry, J. W., and Annis, R. C. (1974). Acculturative stress. *Journal of Cross-Cultural Psychology, 5*, 382–406.

Berry, J. W., Kalin, R., and Taylor, D. M. (1977). *Multiculturalism and Ethnic Attitudes in Canada*. Ottawa: Government of Canada.

Berry, J. W., and Kim, U. (1988). Acculturation and mental health. In P. Dasen, J. W. Berry, and N. Sartorius (eds.), *Health and Cross-Cultural Psychology: Towards Applications*, pp. 207–236. London: Sage.

Berry, J. W., Kim, U., Minde, T., and Mok, D. (1987). Comparative studies of acculturative stress. *International Migration Review, 21*, 491–511.

Berry, J. W., Kim, U., Power, S., Young, M., and Bujaki, M. (1989). Acculturation attitudes in plural societies. *Applied Psychology, 38*, 185–206.

Berry, J. W., Trimble, J., and Olmeda, E. (1986). The assessment of acculturation. In W. J. Lonner and J. W. Berry (eds.), *Field Methods in Cross-Cultural Research*, pp. 291–324. London: Sage.

Canadian Task Force on Mental Health Issues Affecting Immigrants and Refugees (1986). *Review of the Literature on Migrant Mental Health*. Vancouver: University of British Columbia, Department of Psychiatry.

Fozzard, S. (1987). *Mental health and social programmes in closed refugee camps in Hong Kong*. Paper presented at Workshop on Psychological Problems of Refugees and Asylum Seekers, Vitznau, Switzerland.

Graves, T. (1967). Psychological acculturation in a tri-ethnic community. *South-Western Journal of Anthropology, 23*, 337–350.

Honigmann, J. J. (1976). *Personal adaptation as a topic for cultural and social anthropological research*. Chairman's paper, delivered at the Symposium on "The Concept of Adaptation in Studies of American Native Culture Change," American Anthropological Association, Washington, D.C.

Horvath, J. (1987). *Swedish Red Cross Centre Programme for the Rehabilitation of Torture Victims*. Paper presented at Workshop on Psychological Problems of Refugees and Asylum Seekers, Vitznau, Switzerland.

Lam, L. (1987). Prevention of mental health problems in refugees. *Refugee Mental Health Newsletter, 1*, 9–11.

Lazarus, R. S., and Folkman, S. (1984). *Stress, Appraisal and Coping*. New York: Springer.

League of Red Cross and Red Crescent Societies (1986). *Refugees and Displaced Persons in Africa*. Geneva: Author.

League of Red Cross and Red Crescent Societies (1987). *Refugees: The Trauma of Exile*. Dordrecht: Nijhoff.

Murphy, H. B. M. (1965). Migration and the major mental disorders: A reappraisal. In M. B. Kantor (ed.), *Mobility and Mental Health*, pp. 21–43. Springfield, Ill.: Charles C. Thomas.

Rack, P. (1987). *Recent work with elderly refugees in the U.K.* Paper presented at Workshop on Psychological Problems of Refugees and Asylum Seekers, Vitznau, Switzerland.

Redfield, R., Linton, R., and Herskovits, M. J. (1936). Memorandum on the study of acculturation. *American Anthropologist, 38,* 149–152.

Refugee Action (1987). *Report on Seminar on the Psychological Problems of Refugees and Asylum Seekers in the Context of Industrialised Countries.* London: British Red Cross.

Selye, H. (1975). Confusion and controversy in the stress field. *Journal of Human Stress, 1,* 37–44.

Selye, H. (1976). *The Stress of Life,* rev. ed. New York: McGraw-Hill.

Stonequist, E. V. (1937). *The Marginal Man.* New York: Scribner's.

Tyhurst, L. (1980). *Refugee Resettlement.* Paper presented at Second Pacific Congress of Psychiatry, Manila, Philippines.

United Nations High Commission for Refugees (1988). *Guidelines for Working with Refugee Children.* Geneva: Author.

Westermeyer, J. (1986). Migration and psychopathology. In C. L. Williams and J. Westermeyer (eds.), *Refugee Mental Health in Resettlement Countries,* pp. 39–59. Washington, D.C.: Hemisphere.

Westermeyer, J. (1987). Prevention of mental disorder among refugees in the U.S.: Lessons from the period 1976–1986. *Social Science and Medicine, 25,* 941–947.

Williams, C. L. (1987). *Prevention programs in mental health for refugees.* Unpublished paper, University of Minnesota.

World Health Organization (1979). Psychosocial factors and health: New programme directions. In P. Ahmed and G. Coelho (eds.), *Toward a New Definition of Health,* pp. 87–111. New York: Plenum.

3 Child Maltreatment and the Study of Child Refugees

JILL E. KORBIN, Ph.D.

Refugee children are subject to a multitude of harms and threats to their development, well-being, and survival. Whether child refugees are at increased risk of maltreatment relative to other children is an empirical question that has not been answered. The purpose of this chapter is to suggest how the cross-cultural literature on child abuse and neglect might apply to the study of child refugees. The discussion draws primarily on existing literature on cross-cultural child maltreatment rather than on refugees.* The chapter considers definitional issues in cross-cultural child maltreatment research and discusses factors suggested by the cross-cultural record as related to maltreatment. It then turns to a consideration of implications for the study of child maltreatment among refugee children.

DEFINITIONAL ISSUES IN THE CROSS-CULTURAL STUDY OF CHILD MALTREATMENT

"Child abuse" arose as a label of consequence in the United States in the early 1960s. Children with inflicted injuries emerged from the status of an obscure radiological diagnosis (Caffey, 1946) to become a matter of public and professional concern (Adelson, 1961; Elmer, 1960; Kempe, et al., 1962; Nelson, 1984; Pfofl, 1977). When Kempe and colleagues coined the term *the battered child* they referred to a "clinical condition in young children who have received serious physical abuse" (Kempe et al., 1962, p. 17). Since that time, the term *child abuse* has come to refer to a wide range of caretaker acts and child outcomes and encompasses almost anything deemed "bad" for children for which parents or care-

---

*This chapter draws extensively on the author's previously published work on child maltreatment in cross-cultural perspective (Korbin, 1981, 1987a,b).

takers can be held accountable. The breadth of this definition has been detrimental to understanding child maltreatment because the dynamics involved in various forms of maltreatment (e.g., physical, sexual, neglect) do not justify the homogeneous use of the term (e.g., Aber and Zigler, 1981; Giovannoni and Becerra, 1979; Polansky et al., 1981).

Definitional problems are exacerbated in cross-cultural research that addresses comparisons across diverse cultural contexts. Identification of child abuse and neglect in the United States has been based upon identifiable harm to a child which can be attributed to caretaker acts of commission or omission. Neither parental actions nor physical consequences are adequate in and of themselves as critical defining elements of child maltreatment cross-culturally. The same parental behavior may have different meanings and interpretations in different cultural contexts. For example, continual physical contact with an infant is thought to increase chances of survival in societies with high infant mortality, while the same behavior in societies with low infant mortality carries a meaning of indulgence (LeVine, 1977; Super, 1984). Similarly, child outcomes may have different meanings. It does not make sense to equate bruises inflicted by an angry parent with a child who is bruised through the Vietnamese curing practice of *cao gio* (coin rubbing), which is discussed below (Yeatman et al., 1976).

Cross-cultural variability in childrearing beliefs and behaviors suggest that there is not a universal standard for good child care or for child abuse and neglect. This presents a dilemma. Failure to allow for a cultural perspective in defining child abuse and neglect promotes an ethnocentric position in which one's own cultural beliefs and practices are presumed to be preferable, and indeed superior, to all others. Nevertheless, a stance of extreme cultural relativism, in which all judgments of humane treatment of children are suspended in the name of culture, may justify a lesser standard of care for some children. To address this dilemma, definitional issues must be structured into a coherent framework so that child maltreatment can be appropriately identified within and across cultural contexts.

Identification of child maltreatment relies on a complex interaction of (1) harm to the child, (2) caretaker behaviors that produced or contributed to that harm, and (3) societal assignment of culpability or responsibility. Official child abuse and neglect statistics in Euro-American nations reflect harm to a child that resulted in a report to a designated agency. Straus, Gelles, and Steinmetz (1980), in contrast, suggest that attention be addressed to whether behaviors were aggressive and assaultive rather than whether such behaviors result in harm.

Three levels have been suggested for culturally informed definitions of child maltreatment: (1) cultural practices that are viewed as abusive or neglectful from outside the culture, but not by the culture in question; (2) idiosyncratic departure from one's cultural continuum of acceptable behavior; and (3) societally induced harm to children beyond the control of individual parents and caretakers (Korbin, 1981, 1987a). Definitional ambiguity can arise from confusing these three levels. This does not mean that harm at one level is better or worse than harm at another, but it serves to clarify discussion and better inform research and policy.

At the first level, when cultures come into contact, conflict and misunderstanding can occur on a range of issues, including child care patterns and perceptions of child maltreatment. This level is relevant to refugee families who become subject to the standards of the dominant culture of their new country. Most of the literature on child maltreatment among refugees concerns cultural misunderstandings, particularly related to medical practices such as *cao gio* (coin rubbing) among Vietnamese refugees (Feldman, 1984; Gellis and Feingold, 1976; Golden and Duster, 1977; Primosch and Young, 1980; Schmitt, 1988; Yeatman et al., 1976; Yeatman and Viet, 1980). *Cao gio* involves forceful and patterned pushing on the body with a coin. It is intended to drive out illness symptoms of fever, chills, or headaches. The resulting bruises can resemble physical abuse. Children presenting in emergency rooms and clinics with these bruises at first were diagnosed as abused. However, it quickly was recognized that the bruises were inflicted with the intent to help and not harm the child, and *cao gio* is generally excluded from identifications of abuse. Schmitt (1988) lists *cao gio* under "unusual bruises" and notes that the practice should not be confused with child abuse.

Recognition of cultural variability does not necessitate unqualified acceptance of any practice that is cultural. Some cultural practices may be harmful. For example, a form of medicinal substance used to cure *empacho* in children among Hispanics in the Southwest was found to have high concentrations of lead (Trotter et al., 1983). Similar to *cao gio*, the use of this substance is intended to cure illness, not cause harm. Families should not be identified as committing child abuse on the basis of using this substance, even if measures need to be taken to discontinue its use.

The second definitional level involves idiosyncratic departure from cultural standards and norms. All cultures have continua for acceptable and unacceptable child care practices, whether or not the term *maltreatment* is applied. The classically battered, burned, or starved child looks sadly similar across cultural boundaries. The majority of cases of child maltreatment, however, fall into a grey area and require an understanding of the cultural context. The line that separates acceptable from unacceptable childrearing behaviors is often a fine one. For example, despite Sweden's law prohibiting physical punishment, Swedes do not necessarily agree on where the line should be drawn between *aga* (beating) and acceptable discipline (Haeuser, 1982).

Cultural practices may also be misused in a new setting, and may reflect idiosyncratic abuse rather than cultural differences. For example, a newspaper account ("Asian tradition," 1988) reported that the Hmong (a Laotian people) practice of bride capture has been transformed by some into a justification for kidnapping and rape of a desired but unwilling bride. Traditionally, the young groom ritually kidnapped the bride over her culturally required protests. In the traditional context, these culturally prescribed complimentary behaviors were well understood by all participants. The wider network legitimized the union with the exchange of resources signifying marriage. In altered conditions in the United States, however, the misuse of this marriage custom reportedly has resulted in cases of girls being forced against their will into sexual intercourse when they and their families do not consent to marriage.

With respect to the third definitional level of societal abuse and neglect, children around the world are subject to a range of deleterious conditions, including poverty, malnutrition, and armed conflict. The impact of these conditions on children cannot be minimized. These circumstances that affect adults and children alike are generally beyond the control of individual parents or caretakers. However, societal and idiosyncratic maltreatment may overlap. A combination of societal conditions and family dynamics may result in only some children in a family being abused, neglected, or exploited. It is important to determine if some children are more vulnerable to societal harms than others and to consider parental accountability.

THE CULTURAL CONTEXT

A promising contribution of a cross-cultural perspective is an enhanced understanding of the conditions under which child maltreatment is more or less likely to occur. Since regularities in the antecedents and consequences of childrearing practices can be identified cross-culturally (Minturn and Lambert, 1964; Whiting and Whiting, 1975), regularities in the antecedents and consequences of child maltreatment similarly should be amenable to cross-cultural research (Korbin, 1981, 1987b; Levinson, 1989; Rohner, 1975; Scheper-Hughes, 1987). The lack of data specifically on child maltreatment in the cross-cultural record makes postulated causal and outcome factors difficult to identify and analyze. Nevertheless, despite this scarcity of data, the cross-cultural literature on parenting and child care patterns affords an important perspective and suggests future research directions. The following factors have been suggested by the cross-cultural record as potential contributors to abuse.

Categories of Vulnerable Children

In some cultures, it appears that some children are less valued than others. This may be reflected in overt harm to these children or to more covert measures, such as underinvestment or selective neglect (McKee, 1984; Scheper-Hughes, 1985; Scrimshaw, 1978). The cross-cultural record suggests categories of children who are at greater risk of maltreatment (Korbin, 1987b). Some categories, such as gender, can be identified through demographic analyses of differential mortality patterns (Johansson, 1984; Scrimshaw, 1978, 1984), while other categories, such as behavioral and personality characteristics, depend on a thorough understanding of the cultural context. Suggested categories of children at risk should be subjected to further research, both across and within cultures, and do not necessarily apply in all societies. Categories of children who may be at risk include (1) children in poor health or who are malnourished; (2) children who are deformed or handicapped; (3) children who are at developmental stages that are culturally defined as difficult; (4) children whose birth was difficult or unusual (e.g., multiple births); (5) children who are too numerous or too closely spaced and who tax family resources; (6) children with behavioral or personality characteristics that are disvalued in their societies; and (7) children with diminished social supports, such as orphans or stepchildren (Korbin, 1987b).

Social Supports

Even if categories of vulnerable children can be delineated cross-culturally, the potential for maltreatment can be mitigated by social networks. Communities vary in the degree of risk for child maltreatment according to the balance of social supports and stresses (Garbarino and Sherman, 1980). When childrearing is a shared concern within a supportive network, the consequences of having an inadequate or aggressive parent are lessened. The cross-cultural record strongly suggests that children who are embedded in social networks that are supportive in childrearing are less likely to be maltreated. Social support networks serve multiple protective functions for children. First, they provide assistance to parents with child care tasks and responsibilities. Second, networks provide options for the temporary or permanent redistribution of children who may be unwanted in their family of origin. And third, networks afford the context for collective standards, and therefore for the scrutiny and enforcement of parental child care practices (Korbin, 1987b).

Situations of Change

Socioeconomic and sociocultural change has been linked in the literature with an increase in child maltreatment (Gelles and Pedrick-Cornell, 1983; Korbin, 1981; Okeahialam, 1984). Even modest environmental change can impact on child care patterns. For example, some Native American Indian groups initiated harsher and more demanding toilet-training practices following a change from dirt floors, which were easily swept and cleaned, to wooden floors, which required more care (Honigman, 1967). However, the impact of change on child maltreatment is a complex issue. Most often, the literature attributes an increase in child maltreatment to a breakdown in traditional patterns and practices. Change has been associated too readily with a range of social and individual ills, including child maltreatment. This is due, in large part, to a continued reliance on the concept of the folk-urban continuum (Redfield, 1947) that assumes an absence of deviance in traditional, smaller-scale societies. While this assumption of a lack of deviance is not supported by empirical evidence (Edgerton, 1976), the cross-cultural literature suggests that sociocultural and socioeconomic change has an impact on parent-child relationships and interactions, including the potential for maltreatment.

Immigrant and urbanizing families face unique problems that have a potential effect on child maltreatment. In the change from an agrarian to an urban economy, children become consumers rather than producers and an economic liability rather than an asset (LeVine and LeVine, 1985; Logan, 1979; Olson, 1981). Through formal schooling, immigrant children acquire more knowledge of the new environment and society than their parents have and become less obedient and compliant (LeVine and LeVine, 1985), providing greater opportunity for parent-child conflict. Children's behaviors in urban areas are more aggressive and disruptive (Weisner, 1979), and mothers who move to urban areas and come into situations of culture contact are less confident of their efficacy in child rearing (Graves, 1972). These potential problems are exacerbated by increased isolation of families from traditional kin and support networks and diminished availability of sources of support and assistance.

Change can also be positive. In a 20-year perspective on an Indian community, Minturn (1982) found that improvements in locally available medical care promoted the survival and health of female children, thereby diminishing the previous imbalance in the sex ratio. While parents still favored sons and were less willing to transport daughters long distances for medical care, if a clinic was readily accessible, daughters were more likely to receive care than in the past.

IMPLICATIONS FOR THE STUDY OF REFUGEE CHILDREN

Despite their shared experience as children who fled their countries of origin, child refugees are not a homogeneous population and vary along a number of dimensions. Most obviously, child refugees differ according to their culture and nation of origin, to the specific circumstances surrounding their forced relocation, and to the policies and resources of the host country. Child refugees may face very different circumstances based on whether they are alone as unaccompanied minors, with non-related individuals, or with some or all of their family members. Child refugees vary as to the socioeconomic and educational backgrounds they and their families bring to the host country. They differ along the lines of family structure and how well it is suited to the host country. Differences of developmental stage and gender can also affect the experience of refugee children, as they affect the experience of nonrefugee children. These sources of variability must be kept in mind in discussions of maltreatment of refugee children.

In considerations of refugee children and maltreatment, it is important to distinguish among definitional levels. Refugee children suffer a multitude of harms from a number of sources. While not minimizing the harm at any level, it is important for research, service, and policy to recognize its source. These sources may, of course, overlap. First, refugee children may suffer directly from their refugee status. They may suffer from disease, starvation, lack of medical care, and lack of educational opportunities. This corresponds with societal level abuse, but, as noted above, caution is warranted in determining if some children are more vulnerable to harm and if parental culpability is involved. Second, conditions of refugee status such as unemployment, lack of opportunities for parents, or a decreased standard of living in the host country may precipitate or contribute to violence within the family. This corresponds to both societal level and idiosyncratic maltreatment. And third, it must be recognized that children may be idiosyncratically maltreated independent of refugee status and that such maltreatment may result from family dynamics that existed in the prerefugee situation.

Also, as discussed earlier, medical practices of refugees may be misinterpreted by the helping system in the host country. While practices such as *cao gio* have been separated from reportable child abuse incidents, if refugee families are not treated with respect regarding cultural practices, they may not bring their children in for subsequent medical care.

Empirical questions remain: whether refugee children have a higher incidence or prevalence rate of maltreatment, whether they are subject to the same risk factors as nonrefugee children, and whether the circumstances of refugees exacerbate risks of maltreatment by individual caretakers. For example, existing literature on cross-cultural child maltreatment suggests that social networks are a critical factor in protecting children from maltreatment. Determinations could be made regarding the significance of networks among refugees in relation to maltreatment in the indigenous situation, whether the social networks of different groups of refugee children have been diminished, and if so, how they might be replenished.

The concept of *cultural lag,* that is, that all aspects of culture do not change with equal speed and are not equally amenable to alteration, may be relevant to considerations of the impact of change on maltreatment among refugees. Research in some areas, for example, Polynesia, indicates that family and child care patterns are resistant to change (Beaglehole, 1939; Beaglehole and Beaglehole, 1946; Gallimore, Boggs, and Jordan, 1974; Ritchie and Ritchie, 1970). If this is true for groups of refugees, it may afford a buffering for refugee children against various forms of maltreatment.

In discussions of child maltreatment and refugee children, it is important not to lose sight of the individual child and family. Child refugees can be expected to display the range of individual differences seen in other populations, and some may be more resilient than others (e.g., Garmezy and Rutter, 1988). Further, family stress can promote cohesion among members (e.g., in response to illness), as well as precipitate problematic behaviors such as child maltreatment.

CONCLUSION

Despite the scarcity of data, it is reasonable to assume that refugee groups, like other populations, are not immune from child maltreatment. At this juncture, however, it is not possible to make conclusive statements about the incidence, prevalence, etiology, or dynamics of maltreatment among refugee children. It is hoped that this chapter will stimulate further discussion of how the cross-cultural literature on child maltreatment can be applied to improving conditions for refugee children.

REFERENCES

Aber, L., and Zigler, E. (1981). Developmental considerations in the definition of child maltreatment. In R. Rizley and D. Cicchetti (eds.), *Devel-*

opmental Perspectives on Child Maltreatment, pp. 1–29. San Francisco: Jossey-Bass.

Adelson, L. (1961). Slaughter of the innocents. A study of forty-six homicides in which the victims were children. *New England Journal of Medicine, 264,* 1345–1349.

Asian tradition at war with American laws. (1988, February 10). *New York Times,* p. 10.

Beaglehole, E. (1939). *Some Modern Hawaiians.* Honolulu: University of Hawaii Press.

Beaglehole, E., and Beaglehole, P. (1946). *Some Modern Maori.* London: Oxford University Press.

Caffey, J. (1946). Multiple fractures in the long bones of infants suffering from chronic subdural hematoma. *American Journal of Roentgenology, 56,* 163–173.

Edgerton, R. B. (1976). *Deviance: A Cross-Cultural Perspective.* Menlo Park, Calif.: Cummings.

Elmer, E. (1960). Abused young children seen in hospitals. *Social Work, 5,* 98–102.

Feldman, K. (1984). Pseudoabusive burns in Asian refugees. *American Journal of Diseases of Children, 138,* 768–769.

Gallimore, R., Boggs, J. W., and Jordan, C. (1974). *Culture, Behavior and Education. A Study of Hawaiian-Americans.* Beverly Hills, Calif.: Sage.

Garbarino, J., and Sherman, D. (1980). High risk neighborhoods and high risk families: The human ecology of child maltreatment. *Child Development, 51,* 188–198.

Garmezy, N., and Rutter, M. (eds.) (1988). *Stress, Coping, and Development in Children.* Baltimore: Johns Hopkins University Press.

Gelles, R. J., and Pedrick-Cornell, C. (eds.) (1983). *International Perspectives on Family Violence.* Lexington, Mass.: Lexington.

Gellis, S. S., and Feingold, M. (1976). Cao Gio (pseudo-battering in Vietnamese children). *American Journal of Diseases of Children, 130,* 857–858.

Giovannoni, J., and Becerra, R. (1979). *Defining Child Abuse.* New York: Free Press.

Golden, S. M., and Duster, M. C. (1977). Hazards of misdiagnosis due to Vietnamese folk medicine. *Clinical Pediatrics, 16,* 949–950.

Graves, N. (1972). City, country, and child rearing. A tricultural study of mother-child relationships in varying environments. Unpublished Ph.D. dissertation, University of Colorado.

Haeuser, A. (1982). *Sweden's Law Prohibiting Physical Punishment of Children.* Milwaukee: Region V Resource Center on Child Abuse and Neglect.

Honigman, J. (1967). *Personality in Culture.* New York: Harper & Row.

Johansson, S. (1984). Deferred infanticide. Excess female mortality during childhood. In G. Hausfater and S. Hrdy (eds.), *Infanticide: Comparative and Evolutionary Perspectives,* pp. 463–486. New York: Aldine.

Kempe, C. H., Silverman, F. N., Steele, B. F., Droegmueller, W., and Silver, H. K. (1962). The battered child syndrome. *Journal of the American Medical Association, 181,* 17–24.

Korbin, J. E. (ed.) (1981). *Child Abuse and Neglect. Cross-Cultural Perspectives.* Berkeley: University of California Press.

Korbin, J. E. (1987a). Child abuse and neglect. The cultural context. In R. Helfer and C. H. Kempe (eds.), *The Battered Child,* 4th ed., pp. 23–41. Chicago: University of Chicago Press.

Korbin, J. E. (1987b). Child maltreatment in cross-cultural perspective: Vulnerable children and circumstances. In R. Gelles and J. Lancaster (eds.), *Child Abuse and Neglect: Biosocial Dimensions,* pp. 31–35. Chicago: Aldine.

LeVine, R. (1977). Child rearing as cultural adaptation. In P. Leiderman, S. Tulkin, and A. Rosenfeld (eds.), *Culture and Infancy. Variations in the Human Experience,* pp. 15–27. New York: Academic Press.

LeVine, S., and LeVine, R. (1985). Age, gender, and the demographic transition. The life course in agrarian societies. In A. Rossi (ed.), *Gender and the Life Course,* pp. 29–42. New York: Aldine.

Levinson, D. (1989). *Family Violence in Cross-Cultural Perspective.* Beverly Hills, Calif.: Sage.

Logan, R. (1979). Socio-cultural change and the perception of children as burdens. *Child Abuse and Neglect: The International Journal, 3,* 657–62.

McKee, L. (1984). Sex differentials in the survivorship and customary treatment of infants and children. *Medical Anthropology, 8,* 91–108.

Minturn, L. (1982). Changes in the differential treatment of Rajput girls and boys. *Behavior Science Research, 17,* 70–90.

Minturn, L., and Lambert, W. W. (1964). *Mothers of Six Cultures. Antecedents of Childrearing.* New York: Wiley.

Nelson, B. (1984). *Making an Issue of Child Abuse. Political Agenda Setting for Social Problems.* Chicago: University of Chicago Press.

Okeahialam, T. (1984). Child abuse in Nigeria. *Child Abuse and Neglect: The International Journal, 8,* 69–74.

Olson, E. (1981). Socio-economic and psycho-cultural contexts of child abuse and neglect. In J. Korbin (ed.), *Child Abuse and Neglect: Cross-Cultural Perspectives,* pp. 96–119. Berkeley: University of California Press.

Pfofl, S. J. (1977). The "discovery" of child abuse. *Social Problems, 24,* 310–323.

Polansky, N., Chalmers, M., Buttenwieser, E., and Williams, D. (1981). *Damaged Parents. An Anatomy of Child Neglect.* Chicago: University of Chicago Press.

Primosch, R., and Young, S. (1980). Pseudobattering of Vietnamese children (Cao Gio). *Journal of the American Dental Association, 101,* 47–48.

Redfield, R. (1947). The folk society. *American Journal of Sociology, 52,* 293–308.

Ritchie, J., and Ritchie, J. (1970). *Child Rearing Patterns in New Zealand.* Wellington: A. H. and A. W. Reed.

Rohner, R. (1975). *They Love Me, They Love Me Not. A Worldwide Study of the Effects of Parental Acceptance and Rejection.* New Haven, Conn.: HRAF Press.

Scheper-Hughes, N. (1985). Culture, scarcity, and maternal thinking: Maternal detachment and infant survival in a Brazilian shantytown. *Ethos, 13,* 291–317.

Scheper-Hughes, N. (ed.) (1987). *Child Survival. Anthropological Perspectives on the Treatment and Maltreatment of Children.* Dordrecht, Holland: Reidel.

Schmitt, B. D. (1988). Physical abuse. The medical evaluation. In D. Bross, R. Krugman, M. Lenherr, D. Rosenberg, and B. Schmitt (eds.), *The New Child Protection Team Handbook,* pp. 49–65. New York: Garland.

Scrimshaw, S. (1978). Infant mortality and behavior in the regulation of family size. *Population and Development Review, 4,* 383–403.

Scrimshaw, S. (1984). Infanticide in human populations: Societal and individual concerns. In G. Hausfater and S. Hrdy (eds.), *Infanticide: Comparative and Evolutionary Perspectives,* pp. 439–462. New York: Aldine.

Straus, M., Gelles, R., and Steinmetz, S. (1980). *Behind Closed Doors. Violence in the American Family.* New York: Anchor.

Super, C. (1984). Sex differences in infant care and vulnerability. *Medical Anthropology, 8,* 84–90.

Trotter, R., Ackerman, A., Rodman, D., Martinez, A., and Sorvillo, F. (1983). "Azarcon" and "Greta": Ethnomedical solution to epidemiological mystery. *Medical Anthropology Quarterly, 14*(3), 18.

Weisner, T. (1979). Urban-rural differences in sociable and disruptive behavior of Kenya children. *Ethnology, 18,* 153–172.

Whiting, B. B., and J.W.M. Whiting (1975). *Children of Six Cultures. A Psychocultural Analysis.* Cambridge, Mass.: Harvard University Press.

Yeatman, G., Shaw, C., Barlow, M., and Bartlett, G. (1976). Pseudobattering in Vietnamese children. *Pediatrics, 58,* 616–618.

Yeatman, G., and Viet, V. D. (1980). Cao Gio (coin rubbing): Vietnamese attitudes toward health care. *Journal of the American Medical Association, 244,* 2748–2749.

II RESEARCH STUDIES

Research studies focusing on the emotional and social adjustment of refugee children are very limited in number. Given the difficulties and limitations on conducting research on such issues among children generally, this is not a surprising finding. Information is needed on the incidence and prevalence of emotional disturbance among refugee children, in identifying those most at risk, and in assessing the best ways of delivering services to them. Prospective longitudinal studies are especially needed. In this section, four such studies are described, two of which examine the situations of Indochinese children and two of which are devoted to Central American youth.

In Chapter 4, Rubén Rumbaut reports on findings from a survey of Indochinese refugees in San Diego, California, examining the variables influencing adaptation in adults and in their adolescent children. A wide range of variables is assessed for their effects on psychological distress, including, for example, motives for migration, experiences in flight, age, gender, ethnicity, and many others. Students' educational attainment is then related to a series of variables to ascertain patterns of adjustment. This rich study contains a wealth of data and some provocative findings, such as the fact that the youth who are most successful at "becoming American" may be proportionately less successful in academic attainment.

J. David Kinzie and William Sack report in Chapter 5 on a follow-up study of a group of Cambodian adolescents previously found to have many psychiatric problems following exposure to trauma, deprivation, and loss of family members. The study described here documents the long-term effects of massive trauma on children. It also suggests a potential new problem, not previously identified, namely, antisocial behavior for those children who were separated from parents at a very early age such that their early development occurred without a strong attachment figure.

In Chapter 6, Conchita M. Espino describes a study of Central American youth in which the level of exposure to violence prior to arrival in the United States is related to symptomatology for post-traumatic stress disorder and to scores on IQ and achievement tests. Other difficulties experienced by the children in the United States, including poverty and the anxiety of illegal status, were found to add to the difficulties these children have in effecting a healthy and successful adjustment.

4 The Agony of Exile: A Study of the Migration and Adaptation of Indochinese Refugee Adults and Children

RUBÉN G. RUMBAUT, Ph.D.

This chapter reports on findings from a survey of Vietnamese, Cambodian, and Laotian refugees in the San Diego, California metropolitan area, site of one of the largest Indochinese concentrations in the United States. The chapter focuses first on a sample of adult men and women, examining the effects of a wide range of prearrival and postarrival variables on their adaptive responses at two points in time. Next, it moves to a consideration of the adaptation of their adolescent children in San Diego secondary schools, examining the effects of family composition and parental characteristics on the students' educational attainment. Thus, the study does not address the situation of orphaned, unaccompanied, or Amerasian refugee children, but rather that of children who came with one or both parents. They comprise the vast majority of Indochinese children, and for them the family in exile constitutes a central context within which they must forge a new modus vivendi in American schools and communities. Indeed, the Indochinese may now be the youngest population in the United States, with a median age of 18 years (Rumbaut, R. G., 1989a). Hence, the future of these refugee communities in America will depend largely on the mode of incorporation of their children.

THE REFUGEE EXPERIENCE

In the Aftermath of War: Indochinese Refugees in the United States

The Indochinese exodus, a consequence of the longest war of the past two centuries, is one of the largest migrations in modern history. Since the collapse in 1975 of United States–backed regimes in South Vietnam, Cambodia, and Laos, more than 2 million people have fled Indochina in search of asylum elsewhere. Nearly 900,000 of these refugees had been admitted into the United States as of September 30, 1988 (U.S. Committee for Refugees, 1988). Almost two-thirds of them (547,205) have come from Vietnam, and the rest from Laos (192,098) and Cambodia (143,597). A "first wave" of 130,000 people, mostly urban South Vietnamese, were evacuated to the United States in 1975. Most of the refugees, however, began arriving after 1978 as part of a much more heterogeneous "second wave" that peaked in 1980 and has been continuing since. Over 450,000 refugees were resettled in the United States during 1979–1982 alone, and since 1983 the number of Indochinese refugee admissions has stabilized at a rate of approximately 40,000 per year. Despite government policies that have sought to disperse them throughout the 50 states, about 40 percent of the Indochinese population now resides in California. Furthermore, a recent study of their patterns of natural increase estimated that over 200,000 children have been born in the United States to this refugee population (Rumbaut and Weeks, 1986). As a result, the Indochinese as a whole now represent the third largest Asian-origin population in the country, following people of Chinese and Filipino descent—an extraordinary development that has taken place in just over a decade.

A complex set of political and economic factors have shaped the flow of refugees since the end of the Indochina War in 1975. The war shattered the region's economy and traditional society. During the period of U.S. involvement after the defeat of the French at Dien Bien Phu in 1954, it is estimated that over four million Vietnamese soldiers and civilians on both sides were killed or wounded—a casualty rate of nearly 10 percent of the total population. In South Vietnam alone, about a third of the population was internally displaced during the war, and over a half of the total forest area and some 10 percent of the agricultural land was partially destroyed by aerial bombardment, tractor clearing, and chemical defoliation. In Laos the war exacted its greatest toll on the Hmong, an ethnic minority from the rural highlands who had fought on the U.S. side against the Pathet Lao: before the fall of Vientiane about a third of the Hmong population had been uprooted by combat, and their casualty rates were proportionately ten times higher than those of American soldiers in Vietnam. In Cambodia, whose fate was sealed after the expansion of the war in 1970, as many as a quarter of its people may have died during the holocaust of the "killing fields" in the late 1970s. A tragedy of epic proportions, the "war that nobody won" left the countries of the region among the poorest in the world (Isaacs, 1983; Karnow, 1983; Shawcross, 1984).

As is true of refugee movements elsewhere, the first waves of Indochinese refugees were disproportionately comprised of elites who left because of ideological and political opposition to the new regimes, while later flows included masses of people of more modest backgrounds fleeing continuing regional conflicts and deteriorating economic conditions (Portes and Rumbaut, 1990; Rumbaut, R. G., 1989b). Vietnamese professionals and former notables were greatly overrepresented among those who were evacuated to American bases in Guam and the Philippines under emergency conditions during the fall of Saigon; Cambodian and Lao officials and intellectuals, by contrast, were more likely to have gone to France (the former colonial power in Indochina) than to the United States. Among the first to flee on foot across the Mekong river into Thailand were the Hmong, but they were the least likely to be resettled by Western countries at the time; most were to languish in Thai camps for years thereafter. In Vietnam and Laos, meanwhile, it is estimated that hundreds of thousands of persons with ties to the former regimes were interned in "reeducation camps," and in Cambodia the cities were "deurbanized" as the population was forced into labor camps in the countryside. The events of 1975 ensured neither the end of conflict nor exodus from the region.

A massive increase of refugees beginning in late 1978 was triggered by the Vietnamese invasion of Cambodia (which quickly ended three years of Khmer Rouge rule); the subsequent border war between Vietnam and China in 1979 (which accelerated the expulsion of the ethnic Chinese petit bourgeoisie from Vietnam); a new guerilla war in the Cambodian countryside, already wracked by famine and the destruction of the country's infrastructure; and the collapse of both the Chao Fa guerilla resistance against the Pathet Lao and the new system of collective agriculture in Laos, compounded by mismanagement and natural catastrophes. Hundreds of thousands of Cambodian survivors of the Pol Pot labor camps fled to the Thai border along with increased flows of Hmong and other refugees from Laos, and tens of thousands of Chinese and Vietnamese "boat people" attempted to cross the South China Sea packed into rickety crafts suitable only for river travel (many of these sea-going refugees drowned or were assaulted by Thai pirates preying on refugee boats in the Gulf of Thailand). These events led to an international resettlement crisis in 1979 when so-called "first-asylum" countries (principally Thailand, Malaysia, and Indonesia) refused to accept more refugees into their already swollen camps, often forcing refugees in boats back out to sea or forcing land refugees at gunpoint back across border mine fields (U.S. Committee for Refugees, 1984, 1985, 1986; see also Haines, 1985; Mason and Brown, 1983; Strand and Jones, 1985).

In response to the Indochinese refugee crisis, under agreements reached at the Geneva Conference in 1979, Western countries began to absorb significant numbers of the refugee camp population in Southeast Asia. About half of these people have been resettled in the United States (under the provisions of the Refugee Act of 1980), and the rest have been settled primarily in Australia, Canada, and France. Since the early 1980s, harsh "humane deterrence" policies and occasional attempts at forced repatriation have sought to brake the flow of refugees to first-asylum countries, with limited success. During the past decade, an Orderly Departure Program has also allowed the controlled immigration of thousands of Vietnamese directly from Vietnam to the United States. However, by the end of 1988 an estimated 500,000 Indochinese refugees remained in overseas camps, including over 350,000 displaced Cambodians along the Thai border, over 75,000 Laotians in Thailand, and over 70,000 Vietnamese in Hong Kong, Malaysia, Indonesia, Thailand, and the Philippines. About half of these refugees are children. Increasingly, the overseas refugee camp population consists of "long-stayers," reflecting the buildup of people rejected or deemed ineligible for resettlement as well as a new round of arguments among government officials as to whether they are bona fide "political refugees" or "economic migrants" pulled by the perceived opportunity for resettlement in a Western country (U.S. Committee for Refugees, 1989; see also Chan and Loveridge, 1987; Knudsen, 1983; Ressler, Boothby, and Steinbock, 1988; Rosenblatt, 1984).

Sources of Duress and Distress in the Refugee Experience

The literature on migration and mental health has repeatedly observed that long-distance journeys entail stressful life events, at points of both exit and destination, which severely test the emotional resilience of migrants; indeed, the words *travel* and *travail* share a common etymology (Furnham and Bochner, 1986). Although migrants tend to be positively selected relative to nonmigrants and their adaptive resources and responses may vary widely, migration can produce profound psychological distress even among the most motivated and well prepared individuals, and even under the most receptive of circumstances (Rumbaut, R. D., 1977). *Refugees* are typically distinguished from other classes of *immigrants*: the former are viewed as involuntary migrants "pushed" by perceived threats to life or liberty and coercive political conditions, and the latter as voluntary migrants "pulled" by perceived promises of a better future and attractive economic opportunities (David, 1970; Rose, 1981; Stein, 1986; see also Milburn and Watman, 1981). The distinction is in fact more problematic than it seems, since so-called voluntary migrations are not always as voluntary or planned as is claimed, and there are wide differences in the migration experiences of "acute flight" versus "anticipatory" refugees (Kunz, 1973, 1981; Pedraza-Bailey, 1985). Moreover, the status of "refugee" is not self-assigned but rather conferred by host governments for a variety of ideological rather than humanitarian reasons. For example, the official receptions and subsequent adaptation of recent Indochinese "boat people" (deemed bona fide "political" refugees) and Central American escapees (classified as illegal "economic" migrants) reflect such differential labeling, even though both groups have experienced traumatic conditions of persecution and flight (Portes and Rumbaut, 1990).

Since World War II, community surveys of the general population have consistently linked psychological distress to conditions of powerlessness and alienation unbuffered by networks of socioemotional support. Specifically, these studies have reached a consensus on several basic findings: the higher the socioeconomic status, the lower the distress; women and unmarried people are more distressed than men and married people; and the greater the number of undesirable life events, the greater the distress (Mirowsky and Ross, 1986). By implication, the marginal position of many immigrants and refugees is one of relative powerlessness and alienation, affecting their ability to achieve life goals in a foreign world. Further, while both immigrants and refugees must cope with a significant amount of life change, refugees tend to experience more undesirable change, a greater degree of danger, and a lesser degree of control, particularly with respect to the events defining wartorn contexts of exit. Not surprisingly, the recent research literature has repeatedly reported that refugees in general and the Indochinese in particular have experienced greater psychological distress and dysfunction than other immigrant or native-born groups (Baskauskas, 1981; Berry, 1986; Berry et al., 1987; Cohon, 1981; Lin, Tazuma, and Masuda, 1979; Liu, Lamanna, and Murata, 1979; Masuda, Lin, and Tazuma, 1980; Meinhardt et al., 1985–1986; Mollica and Lavelle, 1988; Owan, 1985; Tyhurst, 1951, 1977; Williams and Westermeyer, 1986).

Psychologically, the refugee experience may be conceived as a dialectic of loss and transcendence, entailing a prolonged inner conflict or agony (from the Greek *agonia*, "a struggle or contest for victory," and *agonistes*, "actor"). In the process of acting to reconstruct a meaningful social world in a new country, the resettled refugee is challenged to resolve dual crises: a "crisis of loss"—coming to terms with the past— and a "crisis of load"—coming to terms with the present and immediate future. On the one hand, asylum-seekers are by definition "losers" in sociopolitical conflicts. The refugee loses or is separated from home and homeland, family and friends, work and social status, material possessions, and meaningful sources of identity and self-validation. Refugees from war-torn countries in particular are also often traumatized by violent events prior to and during flight, including life-threatening experiences and the death of significant others. On the other hand, the refugee is overloaded by the compelling pressures to survive, find shelter and work, learn a different language, and adjust to a radically changed environment, often amid conditions of poverty, prejudice, minority status, pervasive uncertainty, and "culture shock" (Furnham and Bochner, 1986; Garza-Guerrero, 1974; Lin, 1986; Oberg, 1960; Stonequist, 1937). The magnitude of the "shock" and the ability to cope with it, in turn, depend on the *social distance* traveled from place of origin to place of destination. Less-educated refugees from rural Southeast Asia clearly have much more difficulty managing the transition to post-industrial American cities than do middle-class migrants of urban origin. Furthermore, in recent years America has been in effect a "moving target" for refugees, requiring not merely adjustments to a new culture but to rapidly changing conditions within the receiving society itself: "culture shock" thus is compounded by "future shock" (Rumbaut and Rumbaut, 1976).

The psychological reaction to these circumstances of exit and entry may entail a long-term process of grief and mourning, heightened anxiety and depression, and an overwhelming sense of helplessness and hopelessness. Survivor guilt and post-traumatic stress disorder have also been observed, notably among catastrophically uprooted Cambodian refugees. On the other hand, although the point is less often noted in the literature oriented toward social pathology, it is also the case that many of the "survivors" beat the odds and excel in their endeavors: mastery of such challenges may deepen a personal sense of efficacy and purpose, enhance the person's energies and productive capacities, and lead to a newfound emancipation (Antonovsky, 1979, 1987; Rumbaut, R. G., 1985; Rumbaut and Rumbaut, 1976). Successful refugees often state that their hardships have made them stronger and built up their sense of self-confidence and self-reliance. While the process of psychological adaptation is thus complex and multidetermined, it is also socially and temporally patterned and predictable (Beiser, 1987, 1988; Portes and Rumbaut, 1990; Rumbaut, R. G., 1989a).

Figure 4.1 presents a general model of the process of migration and adaptation among Indochinese refugees, specifying key antecedent and mediating variables that are hypothesized to influence psychological outcomes over time. The model suggests that the experience of exile is shaped by the interplay of multiple factors, including (1) political, economic, and social contexts of exit and reception; and (2) a variety of prearrival and postarrival individual characteristics. The former include such structural factors as government policies, labor market conditions, and characteristics of ethnic communities at both the points of origin and destination. The latter encompass such variables (which will be described in the section on Migration Motives, below) as the person's

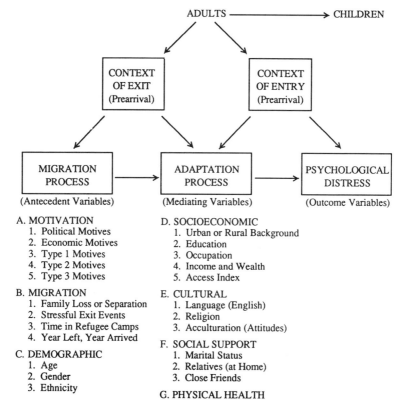

ADULTS ⟶ CHILDREN

CONTEXT
OF EXIT
(Prearrival)

CONTEXT
OF ENTRY
(Prearrival)

MIGRATION
PROCESS
(Antecedent Variables)

ADAPTATION
PROCESS
(Mediating Variables)

PSYCHOLOGICAL
DISTRESS
(Outcome Variables)

A. MOTIVATION
  1. Political Motives
  2. Economic Motives
  3. Type 1 Motives
  4. Type 2 Motives
  5. Type 3 Motives

B. MIGRATION
  1. Family Loss or Separation
  2. Stressful Exit Events
  3. Time in Refugee Camps
  4. Year Left, Year Arrived

C. DEMOGRAPHIC
  1. Age
  2. Gender
  3. Ethnicity

D. SOCIOECONOMIC
  1. Urban or Rural Background
  2. Education
  3. Occupation
  4. Income and Wealth
  5. Access Index

E. CULTURAL
  1. Language (English)
  2. Religion
  3. Acculturation (Attitudes)

F. SOCIAL SUPPORT
  1. Marital Status
  2. Relatives (at Home)
  3. Close Friends

G. PHYSICAL HEALTH

Figure 4.1. Migration, adaptation, and distress: A general model

motives for migration, traumatic events during flight, time spent in refugee camps, year of arrival, age and gender, socioeconomic and cultural background and resources, social supports, and physical and mental health status. The model will be tested with longitudinal data collected by the Indochinese Health and Adaptation Research Project (IHARP) in San Diego, California. A brief description of the project will be presented below, followed by a detailed discussion of results for a probability sample of adult refugees. As is only implied by Figure 4.1, however, the adaptation process—and the meaning and "agony" of exile itself—differ in significant ways for adults and children. These differences among age cohorts and generations deserve further comment.

Refugee Adults and Children: Protagonists and Deuteragonists in Exile

The meaning of exile is differently interpreted by expatriates occupying different generational and socioeconomic positions. When social class is controlled for, parent and youth generations differ in their vantages and modes of response and adaptation. To the parent generation, as the protagonists (from the Greek *protos* and *agonistes,* meaning "first actors") in the decision to leave, exile represents a profound loss and a profound commitment. Their adaptive response typically demands a prolonged mourning of that loss and a vigorous justification of that decision; a lingering sense of the provisionality of their exile and a wish to return to the homeland under new political circumstances ("next year Jerusalem"); a tendency to idealize both the *status quo ante* and the society that offers asylum; and a bitter resistance to any alternative interpretations that may denigrate the meaning of their exile and thus threaten ego integrity. For adults, going into exile is a crucial act of self-definition, and the events of the Indochina War and its aftermath constitute the decisive crisis defining the parent generation of Indochinese refugees. But to the generation of their children, deuteragonists (from *deuteros,* meaning "second") in this drama, exile carries a different relevance and represents less of a vividly felt personal loss than an opaque discontinuity with one's origins, less of a personal commitment than an inherited circumstance. Their adaptive response, sometimes as a reaction formation to perceptions of ethnic discrimination in the receiving society, may too lead to a firm sense of ethnic pride as a source of meaning and identity, but it is essentially devoid of the impulse to justify and protect the parents' world view. The children's generation demands solidarity with the family's common predicament and its perception of a shared crisis, rather than with the particular ideological allegiances of the parent generation; and for the youth the problems of forging new beginnings lack the intense affective significance that this process carries for the adult protagonists who lived the original agony of opting for exile and who are inexorably defined by its consequences. Compared with the children, the refugee adult's time perspective is more focused on the past and the society of origin than on the future and the society of resettlement.

This is not to say, of course, that children are unaffected by their experiences as refugees. Several studies of Indochinese children have identified particular groups at high risk for psychosocial problems (Carlin 1979, 1986; Kinzie et al., 1986; Owan, 1985; Tobin and Friedman, 1984; see also Chapter 5 by Kinzie and Sack in this volume). Of special concern are unaccompanied refugee children who have been separated from their families as a result of wars, natural disasters, or forced migrations. Indeed, a repeated finding of research on children in emergencies over the past 50 years, from the classic work by Anna Freud and Dorothy Burlingham during World War II to more recent crises, is that the *separation* of children from their parents, no matter how purposeful and well intentioned, is more traumatic to children than their actual exposure to bombings and the witnessing of destruction, injury, and death. Studies of children who have experienced emigration, expulsion from their homeland, traumatic flight, refugee camps, and even concentration camps have found that those who remained with their parents (or surviving parent) showed much less psychological disturbance than those who had been separated from their families while enduring the same events (for a thorough review of this literature, see Ressler, Boothby, and Steinbock, 1988). In fact, as a general rule, the *shared* experience of crisis tends to increase family cohesiveness and morale; family bonds are more likely to be strengthened rather than disrupted as members close ranks for mutual security in response to a common threat. However differently it may be defined by refugee parents and their children, it is precisely the shared circumstance of exile that creates a singular bond between them, a source of solidarity and mutual confirmation (Rumbaut, R. G., 1976).

In general, however, children adjust much more rapidly and flexibly than adults to a new society—for example, they learn the new language relatively quickly and without an accent, and are more likely to pick up new customs as well—often leading to parent-child conflict and an "adaptation lag" between the old and the young that may widen the "generation gap" more familiar to the native-born (Rumbaut and Rumbaut, 1976). These differences are most clearly apparent between foreign-born adult refugees and their U.S.-born offspring. Between these two groups, however, is a group of refugee youth that differs in still other ways. Children who were born abroad but are being educated and come of age in the United States form what may be called the "1.5" generation. These refugee youth must cope with two crisis-producing and identity-defining life transitions: (1) adolescence and the task of managing the transition from childhood to adulthood, and (2) acculturation and the task of managing the transition from one sociocultural environment to another. The "first" generation of their parents, who are fully part of the "old" world, face only the latter; the "second" generation of children now being born and reared in the United States, who as such become fully part of the "new" world, will need to confront only the former. But members of the "1.5" generation form a distinctive cohort in that in many ways they are marginal to both the old and the new worlds, and are fully part of neither of them. Still they need to search for an identity and define themselves with respect both to their society of origin, to which they may never return, and to the adoptive society where they are being formed, which is itself rapidly changing.

In this sense, the generation of "1.5ers" share and must adapt within a common psychohistorical actuality. We will examine the adaptation of this group of refugee youth later in this chapter.

THE ADULTS

The IHARP Study: Sample and Sources of Data

The IHARP study collected survey data at two points in time a year apart—T1 (1983) and T2 (1984)—through in-depth interviews with a probability sample of Indochinese refugees (for details, see Rumbaut, R. G., 1989a). The interviews were conducted in the home and language of the respondents by trained coethnic interviewers and encompassed complete migration and resettlement histories, including social background characteristics, family composition and change, and longitudinal measures of English language proficiency, training, employment, income, social support, physical health, and mental health status. The sample is representative of an Indochinese population universe systematically enumerated at nearly 40,000 as of April 1983 in San Diego County, California. Universe enumeration lists were developed for each of the five major Indochinese ethnic groups—Vietnamese, Chinese-Vietnamese, Cambodian (Khmer), Hmong, and Lao—and from them simple random samples were drawn. If the adult respondent selected in the sample was married, the spouse was also (separately) interviewed.

The resulting T1 sample includes 739 adults from the five major groups, ranging in age from 18 to 71 years old. The sample contains approximately equal numbers of men (366) and women (373). The 739 respondents in the T1 sample resided in 437 households containing 3,003 persons overall. The Lao sample ($N = 140$), however, was interviewed only at T1; we only have cross-sectional data for the Lao. T1 to T2 longitudinal data are thus available only for the Vietnamese, Chinese, Cambodian, and Hmong ($N_{T1} = 599$; $N_{T2} = 500$). The resulting T2 sample contains 252 women and 248 men. Difference-of-means tests were conducted to compare the demographic, socioeconomic, health, and mental health characteristics of the 99 persons who could not be reinterviewed at T2 against the 500 who were interviewed at both T1 and T2. The results show no statistically significant differences between them. This evidence suggests that sample attrition produced no significant bias in the follow-up sample. Thus, findings from the T2 sample remain validly generalizable to the population universes from which they were drawn. Given our interest in this chapter in examining the adaptation of these respondents over time, we will rely on the T1 to T2 longitudinal adult sample ($N = 500$) for the analyses that follow.

Table 4.1. Measuring Psychological Distress among Indochinese Refugees at T1 (1983) and T2 (1984)

Psychological Distress Scale	Mean Scores[a]		Factor Loadings	
Q: How often in the past month have you:	T1	T2	T1	T2
1. Felt sad, discouraged, hopeless, worthless?	1.66	1.53	.737	.745
2. Felt down-hearted and blue?	1.57	1.46	.706	.750
3. Felt under strain, stress, pressure?	1.44	1.41	.747	.752
4. Felt anxious, worried, upset?	1.70	1.60	.680	.788
5. Been thinking of some things all the time?	1.78	1.63	.667	.724
6. Had trouble keeping your mind on activity?	2.03	1.80	.642	.644
7. Been bothered by nervousness or "nerves"?	1.51	1.38	.512	.638
8. Felt tired, worn out, used up, exhausted?	1.40	1.40	.597	.600
Total 8-item Distress Scale Score	1.64	1.53		

Source: IHARP Longitudinal Adult Sample (see, e.g., Rumbaut, R. G., 1985, 1989a,b; Rumbaut and Weeks, 1986; Rumbaut et al., 1988).

[a]Mean scores are interpretable on a 0–5 scale, where 5 = constantly (all of the time), 4 = very often (most of the time), 3 = often, 2 = sometimes, 1 = rarely, and 0 = never, as reported by the respondent at interviews a year apart (T1 and T2) for distress symptoms experienced over the past month. The eight items composing the distress scale were identified through factor analysis (VARIMAX rotation) of a larger battery of psychological well-being items. Factor loadings are given for the items clustering on the principal component (distress factor), which accounted for 40% of the variance in the sample. Two lesser factors (reflecting euphoric and somatic symptoms) were identified by the analysis but are not here considered.

Measuring Psychological Distress

The psychological adaptation of the adult sample was measured by a widely used screening scale, the General Well-Being Index (GWB), developed and validated by the National Center for Health Statistics in the 1970s (Link and Dohrenwend, 1980; Rumbaut, R. G., 1985, 1989a). This scale contains indicators of the frequency of affective symptoms experienced by the respondent over the past month. A factor analysis of these items revealed the presence of three principal components. Eight items loaded above a 0.50 criterion on the main factor, accounting for 40 percent of the variance. These items, listed in Table 4.1, reflect dysphoric symptoms and a sad, anxious, and depressed mood; taken together they compose the measure of psychological distress we will employ in the discussion that follows. (The other two factors identified by the analysis reflected euphoric and somatic symptoms, respectively; we will not be concerned with them here.) The eight-item distress measure showed a high degree of internal consistency; reliability coefficients (Cronbach's alpha) were 0.834 at T1 and 0.873 at T2, a noteworthy result

Table 4.2. Psychological Distress Scores by Ethnicity and Gender

Psychological Distress Scores by Ethnicity and Gender:	TIME (T1/T2)	Hmong (N= 109)	Khmer (N= 120)	Chinese (N= 114)	Vietnamese (N= 157)	Total (N= 500)
Female (N=252)	T1	1.85	2.06	1.42	1.36	1.66
	T2	1.71	1.97	1.53	1.46	1.66
Male (N=248)	T1	1.92	2.31	1.23	1.23	1.62
	T2	1.49	1.83	1.32	1.10	1.39
Total	T1	1.88	2.18	1.33	1.29	1.64
	T2	1.60	1.90	1.43	1.25	1.53

Source: IHARP Longitudinal and Adult Sample (see, e.g., Rumbaut, R. G., 1985, 1989a,b; Rumbaut and Weeks, 1986; Rumbaut et al., 1988).

in view of the ethnocultural diversity of the Indochinese respondent groups.

Table 4.2 also presents distress scores at T1 and T2 for the sample as a whole, and by gender and ethnicity. Overall, there was a decrease in distress symptoms between T1 and a year later at T2. There was no significant difference between men and women at T1, but by T2 men reflected considerable improvement while the psychological status of women remained essentially unchanged. This finding matches those of other studies that have consistently reported greater levels of distress among women. At both time periods, the Cambodians (Khmer) exhibited the highest distress scores, followed by the Hmong, the Chinese-Vietnamese, and the Vietnamese. As expected, although not shown in Table 4.2, significantly higher distress scores were also found for refugees who had suffered a greater degree of family loss or separation and who had spent the longest time in refugee camps overseas, respondents over 50 years of age, persons of rural background, the least educated and English-proficient, and the unemployed. Lower distress scores were found for those who were married and who had more relatives and close friends nearby, indicating the buffering effects of social support. Following the model outlined earlier in Figure 4.1, these characteristics of the migration and adaptation process will be described below, broken down by ethnic group and gender. A multivariate analysis will then be presented to sort out and specify the independent effects on psychological distress of all such predictor variables.

Migration Motives

We noted above that the distinction often made between refugees and other classes of immigrants revolves around their different motives for migration and the traumatic nature of their flight experiences. In particular, refugees are said to be motivated to flee by fear of persecution ("political" motives), while immigrants are defined by their aspirations for better material opportunities and self-advancement ("economic" motives). Despite the importance of motivational variables, however, scarcely any systematic studies in the research literature have focused on this topic. The debate on these matters has thus been governed more by assumptions and impressions than hard evidence. At the T1 interviews, respondents were asked to state all of their motives for leaving the homeland, and these were then coded and quantified. What emerged was a complex picture: over 50 different reasons were given, ranging from fear of repression or imprisonment in reeducation camps, to past associations with the former regime and ideological opposition to communism, to desires for family reunification, better education for their children, and an improved standard of living. Some of these reasons may be categorized as "political" in nature, others as "economic" or "social." Often both types of reasons were cited by the same respondent, making the usual distinction between refugees and non-refugees overly simplistic and misleading, and suggesting that political and economic considerations may be inextricably linked or additive rather than mutually exclusive zero-sum motivations. Moreover, the respondents clearly differed in the degree of "motivational duress" that they experienced—that is, the degree of perceived danger and lack of control over threatening events that set in motion their decision to leave. Put differently, refugees vary in the degree to which they reflect the stereotype; being a refugee is not a motivationally homogeneous phenomenon.

To clarify the diversity of reported motives, a factor analysis was conducted and the data were reduced to a set of six main types of exit motives. A typology of these motives is detailed in Table 4.3. Of the six main types of reasons identified, three involved "political" (type A) motivations: (1A) specific perceptions of fear or force, (2A) past political associations or generalized fear, and (3A) ideological reasons; the other three types involved more "socioeconomic" (type B) considerations: (1B) harsh material conditions of famine and poverty, (2B) loss of personal property or wealth, and (3B) miscellaneous "pull" motives, such as seeking a better future or family reunification. The typology in Table 4.3 also classifies these six types of motives according to their degree of

Table 4.3. A Typology of Migration Motives and Their Correlations with Postarrival Distress at T1 (1983) and T2 (1984)

| Type & Time | Motivational Duress (Degree of Perceived Danger and Lack of Control in Decision to Leave) | | | |
| | Higher | | Lower | |
	1	2	3	Σ
A	Force or Fear (1A)[a]	Past assns. (2A)[b]	Ideological (3A)[c]	"Political"
T1	.363	.086	−.125	.321
T2	.193	.041	−.080	.156
B	Harsh or Poor (1B)[d]	Property lost (2B)[e]	"Pull" motives (3B)[f]	"Economic"
T1	.219	.094	−.055	.189
T2	.125	.018	−.011	.101
Σ	Motive—type 1	Motive—type 2	Motive—type 3	
T1	.361	.124	−.137	
T2	.194	.040	−.070	

Source: IHARP Longitudinal and Adult Sample, N=500.

[a]1A: Force/fear = forced relocation, forced to new economic zone, forced into a reeducation camp, imprisoned prior to exit; specific fear of harm from new regime, fear of arrest, fear of communists, fear of future.

[b]2A: Past assns. = past association with American military, Central Intelligence Agency (CIA), government; past political involvement with old regime, armed forces; drafted to fight in Kampuchea; general harassment; generalized fear.

[c]3A: Ideological = seeking freedom; hatred, dislike of communists; protesting present conditions; refusal to join a cooperative; stranded in United States in April 1975; other political-ideological reasons.

[d]1B: Harsh/poor = starvation, famine, lack of food, harsh or poor economic conditions; hard work, no rewards, inability to make a living.

[e]2B: Property lost = loss or confiscation of personal or income-producing property or wealth or both.

[f]3B: "Pull" motives = seeking better future, better education; to reunify with family members abroad; given opportunity to leave; persuaded by family or friends to leave; other miscellaneous reasons.

"motivational duress." Thus, along a duress continuum three main types of motives can be identified: those involving a high degree of duress (types 1A + 1B), intermediate (types 2A + 2B) and relatively lower levels of duress (types 3A + 3B). An index of each of these three latter types was composed by summing all respective motives to form the measures labeled in Table 4.3 as "type 1," "type 2," and "type 3" motives.

Table 4.3 also presents correlations among these various exit motive indices and the level of postarrival psychological distress measured at both T1 and T2. The results suggest that the greater the motivational duress at the point of exit, the greater the level of psychological distress at the point of destination. Strong positive correlations with distress were noted for refugees reporting type 1 (high-duress) motives: fear or force experiences (1A) and harsh or poor conditions (1B). Weak positive correlations with distress were noted for type 2 motives: past associations (2A) and property lost (2B). Type 3 motives were *negatively* correlated with distress: ideological reasons (3A) and socioeconomic "pull" motives (3B). Ideological motives actually reflected the most negative associations with psychological distress, suggesting a greater degree of "cognitive control" in the decision to leave that is more characteristic of upper social classes and less characteristic of the experiences of lower-class refugees who were also more likely to report starving or directly fearing for their lives as their reasons for flight.

Moreover, as Table 4.4 shows, there are statistically significant differences among ethnic groups in each of these six motive indices. Cambodians reported the most type 1 motives (reflecting their life-threatening experiences during the Pol Pot period of the late 1970s) as well as both more "political" *and* "economic" exit motives. The Hmong reported more type 2 motives, the Vietnamese more ideological motives, and the Chinese more economic "pull" motives as well as the fewest past associations with the former regime. Men reported significantly more political motives than women—suggesting that women were less likely than men to have controlled the decision to leave—but there were no differences by gender with respect to economic motivations. Despite this diversity of motives in the refugees' decision to leave, by far more fear or force motives were reported overall (2.22) than any of the other five motive types; loss or confiscation of property ranked next in reported frequency (0.79), followed by ideological reasons (0.56), harsh or poor conditions (0.52), "pull" motives (0.38), and lastly past associations and generalized fear (0.28). By this classification, more "political" (3.05) than "economic" (1.68) motives were reported, providing at least some support to the oft-used phenomenological definition of the refugee experience.

Migration Events

Other variables defining the exit experiences of the refugee sample are broken down in Table 4.4 by ethnicity and gender. One is a measure of family loss and separation—composed of such variables as deaths and imprisonment of close family members, escape alone, and inability to locate or communicate with family members left behind. Clearly, the Cambodians suffered the greatest number of family loss and separation events—two-thirds of this population reported the death of one or more

Table 4.4. Characteristics of the Indochinese Migration Process, by Ethnicity and Gender

Migration Variables	Hmong (N = 109)	Khmer (N = 120)	Chinese (N = 114)	Vietnamese (N = 157)
Migration motives[b]				
Motives—type 1	2.71	5.40	1.54	1.58
Force or fear motives (1A)	2.56	3.65	1.39	1.48
Harsh/poor conditions (1B)	0.15	1.75	0.16	0.10
Motives—type 2	1.29	0.88	0.96	1.13
Past govt. assns. (2A)	0.33	0.33	0.16	0.30
Property or wealth lost (2B)	0.96	0.56	0.80	0.83
Motives—type 3	0.56	0.93	1.14	1.04
Ideological motives (3A)	0.35	0.54	0.60	0.68
"Pull" motives (3B)	0.21	0.39	0.54	0.35
"Political" motives	3.24	4.52	2.14	2.46
"Economic" motives	1.32	2.70	1.50	1.27
Migration events				
Family loss or separation[c]	2.59	4.45	2.10	2.28
% Family member died	59.6	65.8	32.5	39.5
% Family member in prison	7.3	2.5	12.3	40.1
% Fled alone without family	19.3	29.2	11.4	13.4
% No family communication (whereabouts unknown)	12.8	61.7	12.3	3.8
Exit events reported[d]	4.46	5.14	4.74	5.64
Exit events—type 1	2.47	3.08	1.88	2.12
Exit events—type 2	0.31	0.46	0.32	0.37
Exit events—type 3	1.68	1.60	2.54	3.15
Months in refugee camps	34.4	25.8	10.4	7.4
Time and age				
Year left homeland (19___)	76.4	77.8	78.6	78.3
Year arrived in United States (19___)	79.3	80.3	79.5	78.9
Age at arrival (years)	33.4	32.9	38.7	32.1

Source: IHARP Longitudinal and Adult Sample, N=500.

Abbreviations: NS, not significant.

[a]Significance (p) of differences among groups: **p < .01, *p < .05.

[b]Measures are composite indices of types of motives reported. See Table 4.3 for variables comprising each motive index.

[c]Measure is a composite index of the following variables: death of spouse, children, and other close family members; escaped alone without immediate family; separated from and cannot now communicate with family members; family members now imprisoned.

close relatives, and over 60 percent still did not know and had no way of knowing the whereabouts of family members left behind in Cambodia—followed by the Hmong and the Vietnamese. The Chinese were most likely to have left together as a family, a fact that is partly reflected

p^a	Male (N = 248)	Female (N = 252)	p^a	Total (N = 500)
**	2.87	2.60	NS	2.73
**	2.38	2.06	*	2.22
**	0.49	0.55	NS	0.52
**	1.20	0.94	**	1.07
*	0.40	0.17	**	0.28
**	0.81	0.77	NS	0.79
**	0.98	0.89	NS	0.93
**	0.64	0.48	**	0.56
**	0.34	0.41	NS	0.38
**	3.40	2.70	**	3.05
**	1.63	1.72	NS	1.68
**	2.82	2.83	NS	2.83
**	48.4	48.8	NS	48.6
**	18.9	16.3	NS	17.6
**	23.0	13.1	**	18.0
**	21.8	21.4	NS	21.6
NS	5.09	5.02	NS	5.06
**	2.33	2.42	NS	2.37
NS	0.37	0.36	NS	0.37
**	2.40	2.23	NS	2.32
**	18.0	18.8	NS	18.4
**	77.7	77.9	NS	77.8
**	79.3	79.7	NS	79.5
**	34.7	33.5	NS	34.1

[d]Exit events is a composite index of three types of stressful events reported during the migration process: Events—type 1 include: feared would be killed during escape; robbed, assaulted, shot at; went without food or water; witnessed violent deaths during flight. Events—type 2 include: was ill, injured, wounded, or pregnant during flight. Events—type 3 include: gave bribes to exit; boat sunk; boat engine broke down; not allowed to land; expelled; shipwrecked; picked up, towed, rescued at sea.

in their older age overall. These loss or separation events did not differ significantly by gender, although men were more likely than women to have fled alone.

During the process of flight, the respondents were also exposed to a wide range of traumatic events. Three main types of such events were identified through factor analysis, described as "exit events" in Table 4.4. There were no significant differences by gender in the number or type of exit events reported—both men and women went through similar flight experiences—although as "boat people," the experiences of the Chinese and Vietnamese clearly differed from those of the Hmong and Cambodian land refugees. Once they reached a country of first asylum, Table 4.4 shows that the Hmong stayed in refugee camps far longer than any other group before being resettled in the United States, followed by the Cambodians, the Chinese, and the Vietnamese. Data on their average year of departure and of arrival are also provided in Table 4.4. The Cambodians are the most recent arrivals in the United States, while the Vietnamese as a group have been here the longest (reflecting the fact that most 1975 "first-wave" refugees were Vietnamese). There were no significant differences by gender on any of these latter aspects of the migration process.

The Adaptation Process

On arrival in the United States, a decisive factor governing the refugees' adaptation process is their social class of origin. As Table 4.5 shows, over a third of the refugee sample came from rural backgrounds in Southeast Asia. However, about 90 percent of the Hmong and 55 percent of the Cambodians came from rural areas, while the Chinese and Vietnamese were overwhelmingly from urban sectors in South Vietnam. These differences are reflected in their levels of premigration education: the Vietnamese were the most educated (9.8 years), followed by the Chinese (6.6 years), the Cambodians (4.9 years), and the Hmong (1.7 years). In each ethnic group, men were significantly more educated than women, indicating the subordinate status of women in the society of origin. Although not shown in Table 4.4, first-wave refugees were much more likely to come from highly educated professional and managerial classes, while more recent arrivals are less educated farmers, fishers, and manual laborers. Vietnamese and Hmong men included high proportions of former military officers and soldiers, while the ethnic Chinese—a largely segregated "middleman" minority of merchants from the Cholon area of Saigon—were least likely to have had any prior involvement with either the army of the Republic of Vietnam (ARVN) or the South Vietnamese or American governments during the war. This was implied previously in the fact that few Chinese-Vietnamese cited "past associations" in their motives to flee. The Hmong were primarily preliterate peasants, and their language lacked an alphabet until the 1950s when missionaries in Laos developed a written notation for their language, which had been exclusively oral until that time (Rumbaut, R. G., 1989b).

These background characteristics are in turn reflected in the refugees' socioeconomic position at T1 and T2. The same ethnic group rank order is mirrored in their levels of employment and labor force participation in the San Diego economy, although all groups are progressing gradually if at different rates over time. Indochinese women had more children than American women and were much less likely to be active participants in the labor force (Rumbaut and Weeks, 1986). Most refugee families reported very low annual incomes, and indeed by T2 about 75 percent of the families in the sample had incomes that fell below the federal poverty line. Another revealing socioeconomic indicator of their ability to meet basic needs is a composite measure of problems experienced by the respondents in accessing health care services (see Table 4.5). These included language, transportation, and other barriers. In each of these, highly significant differences are again apparent by ethnic group and gender (Rumbaut et al., 1988).

Two types of indicators of cultural adaptation are presented in Table 4.5: a measure of English language reading and writing proficiency, and three items measuring attitudes toward acculturation on an agree-disagree response scale. English literacy gradually increases over time; it is primarily a function of level of education, and secondarily of (younger) age and longer time of residence in the United States. The three attitudinal items listed in Table 4.5 were worded as follows: (1) "The schools should help our children learn American ways of behaving and become more like the American children in the neighborhood"— an indicator of *assimilationism*; (2) "We may adapt ourselves to American society in order to earn a living, but we must stay together as a group to preserve our own culture"—an indicator of *biculturalism*; and (3) "The American way of life may be good for others, but not for me"—an indicator of *traditionalism*. In all three there are significant differences by ethnic group but not by gender, except that men are more likely than women to seek a bicultural adaptive strategy.

Finally, Table 4.5 provides data on marital status and other social support variables, and an objective measure of physical health status. Most of the adults in the sample (87 percent) were married, and divorce (which is highly stigmatized in these Asian communities) was rare. Over 20 percent of Cambodian women were widowed, however, reflecting the high death rates of the late 1970s. More Vietnamese and Cambodians were single than the Chinese or the Hmong. None of the Hmong were single, and they lived in the most crowded households. Cambodians also lived in large households, though many of the boarders were not family members. As would be expected, close friends were mainly

Table 4.5. Characteristics of the Indochinese Adaptation Process, by Ethnicity and Gender

Adaptation Variables	Hmong (N = 109)	Khmer (N = 120)	Chinese (N = 114)	Vietnamese (N = 157)
Socioeconomic				
Education (years)	1.7	4.9	6.6	9.8
% Rural origin	89.9	55.0	4.4	5.1
% Employed (T1)	17.4	16.7	21.1	35.7
% Employed (T2)	18.4	21.7	30.7	46.5
% Not in labor force (T1)	65.1	76.7	64.9	42.0
% Not in labor force (T2)	64.2	70.8	61.4	40.1
% Below poverty line (T1)[b]	93.3	82.3	81.3	57.0
% Below poverty line (T2)	88.3	81.0	76.6	61.3
Annual family income (T1)[b]	8,809	7,725	8,315	11,574
Annual family income (T2)	9,876	8,118	9,150	12,163
Health Access Problem Index[c]	3.9	3.2	2.1	1.2
% Language problem	82.6	85.0	53.5	28.0
% Worry MediCal cutoff	84.4	71.7	70.2	46.5
% Transportation problem	56.0	68.3	27.2	11.5
% Services too far away	51.4	25.8	21.1	3.8
% Too long wait	72.5	30.0	22.8	26.8
% No help received	22.0	19.2	8.8	1.9
Acculturation				
English literacy index (T1)[d]	1.07	1.11	1.18	2.02
English literacy index (T2)	1.35	1.37	1.42	2.28
Item 1 (learn American way)[e]	5.54	2.71	4.76	4.94
Item 2 (adapt but keep culture)	5.36	5.06	4.89	5.00
Item 3 (American way not good)	3.38	3.84	3.25	3.28
Social support				
% Married	95.4	74.2	91.2	87.3
% Single	0	11.7	5.3	12.1
% Widowed	2.8	11.7	2.6	0.6
% Divorced, separated	1.8	2.5	0.9	0
No. relatives at home[b]	9.0	6.0	5.4	4.9
No. close coethnic friends	4.4	2.5	3.4	3.7
No. close American friends	0.8	0.6	0.8	0.9
Physical health				
QWB (1.0 = optimum health)[f]	0.836	0.907	0.840	0.913

Source: IHARP Longitudinal Adult Sample, N = 500.

Abbreviations: NS, not significant.

[a]Significance (*p*) of differences between groups: **$p < .01$; *$p < .05$.

[b]Data reported by family, not by individual (N = 296 households, including 48 female-headed households).

[c]Measure is a composite index of health care access problems specified below in the table.

[d]Index of English reading and writing proficiency, on scale of 0 = none, 1 = poor, 2 = some, 3 = fair, 4 = good, 5 = fluent.

p^a	Male (N = 248)	Female (N = 252)	p^a	Total (N = 500)
**	7.4	4.8	**	6.1
**	34.3	36.5	NS	35.4
**	31.9	15.9	**	23.8
**	41.5	20.2	**	30.8
**	39.9	81.0	**	60.6
**	37.5	77.4	**	57.6
**	74.2	87.5	*	76.4
**	73.8	83.3	*	75.3
**	9,996	5,642	**	$9,297
**	10,642	6,487	**	$9,968
**	1.9	3.0	**	2.5
**	50.4	68.3	**	59.4
**	58.1	74.2	**	66.2
**	26.2	50.4	**	38.4
**	14.1	32.5	**	23.4
**	25.8	47.2	**	36.6
**	8.1	15.9	**	12.0
**	1.70	1.11	**	1.40
**	1.96	1.37	**	1.66
**	4.48	4.50	NS	4.49
**	5.15	4.98	*	5.07
*	3.50	3.36	NS	3.43
**	87.5	86.1	NS	86.8
**	11.3	4.4	**	7.8
**	0	8.3	**	4.2
**	1.2	1.2	NS	1.2
**	6.3	5.0	*	6.1
**	4.0	2.9	**	3.5
NS	0.9	0.6	*	0.8
**	0.906	0.851	**	0.878

[e]Attitude items measured at T1 on a seven-point scale from 0 = strongly disagree to 6 = strongly agree. See text for wording of items.

[f]Score on Quality of Well-Being (QWB) Scale, an objective measure of physical health composed of weighted physical symptoms and health-related dysfunctions experienced by respondent over previous 6 days.

coethnics rather than Americans. Men reported more close friends, both coethnic and American, than women—reflecting the general restriction of the refugee women to the home and their relative isolation from the workplace and the larger community. The Vietnamese and men generally reflected better physical health (based on the Quality of Well-Being [QWB] Scale, a composite measure of physical symptoms and health-related dysfunctions experienced by the respondent over the previous 6 days). Lower physical health scores were exhibited by the Hmong, the Chinese (who are older), and women generally.

Determinants of Psychological Distress

Although the above portrait of aspects of the refugee adaptation process is selective, it reveals considerable complexity and variation. All of those variables may be interrelated, and all may variously influence psychological well-being or distress over time. To clarify such associations, a zero-order correlation matrix is presented in Table 4.6 for variables that were tested in multiple regression analyses of distress. A few points seem worth highlighting. With respect to migration motives, type 1 motives are not associated with either type 2 or type 3 motives, but they are strongly correlated with greater family loss, longer time in refugee camps, and lower socioeconomic status. Type 3 motives are modestly associated with less time in the camps and higher socioeconomic status. The more recent the year of arrival, the lower the socioeconomic status and the level of English proficiency, and the fewer the number of close friends. The index of health access problems is strongly correlated with lower socioeconomic status, poor English, and poor physical health. The younger the age at arrival, the better the level of English competency and physical health. Of the items measuring acculturation attitudes, item 1 (assimilationism) is negatively associated with type 1 motives and family loss, but item 2 (biculturalism) and item 3 (traditionalism) are not significantly correlated with other variables. Of the social support indicators, the number of relatives in households is greater among the most socially isolated (rural-origin refugees with little education and poor command of English), while the number of close friends is greater for persons who are least isolated (those who are employed, are more English-proficient, have higher incomes, and have lived a longer time in the United States). Most of the 21 independent variables listed in the matrix show statistically significant correlations with distress outcomes at both T1 and T2. For an ordinary least-squares regression procedure, two variables in Table 4.6 posed multicollinearity problems: education and English literacy. For this reason, they are not included in the regression models presented below.

Table 4.6. Intercorrelations of Migration, Adaptation, and Psychological Distress Variables

No.	Variable	1	2	3	4	5	6	7	8	9	10	11	12	13	14	15	16	17	18	19	20	21	22
1.	Motive—type 1	1.00																					
2.	Motive—type 2	.05	1.00																				
3.	Motive—type 3	-.10	-.15	1.00																			
4.	Family loss	.36	.00	.05	1.00																		
5.	Time in camps	.25	-.01	-.18	.06	1.00																	
6.	Migration events	.12	.11	-.02	.11	-.03	1.00																
7.	Year of arrival	.33	-.07	.03	.10	.32	.14	1.00															
8.	Rural origin	.30	.03	-.21	.11	.57	-.04	.16	1.00														
9.	Education	-.18	.08	.17	-.11	-.52	.02	-.33	-.57	1.00													
10.	English literacy	-.15	.12	.06	-.08	-.32	-.01	-.38	-.33	.72	1.00												
11.	Access index	.27	-.02	-.19	.19	.44	.03	.29	.46	-.55	-.49	1.00											
12.	Not in labor force	.04	-.10	-.09	.01	.24	-.02	.24	.21	-.48	-.46	-.22	1.00										
13.	Family income	-.22	.03	.04	-.09	-.22	-.05	-.54	-.18	.35	.39	-.32	.42	1.00									
14.	Accult.—item 1	-.43	.11	-.01	-.33	-.04	.03	-.10	-.00	-.06	-.02	-.08	.06	.04	1.00								
15.	Accult.—item 2	.03	.02	-.05	.04	.09	.03	-.10	.17	-.10	-.03	.09	-.04	.06	.03	1.00							
16.	Accult.—item 3	.11	.04	-.06	.09	.04	.07	.06	.05	-.03	.03	.14	.00	-.02	-.03	.16	1.00						
17.	Married	-.13	.09	-.07	-.24	-.00	.05	-.09	-.09	-.05	-.07	-.03	.08	.19	.11	-.04	-.05	1.00					
18.	Relatives	.08	.01	-.08	-.12	.28	-.07	-.06	.36	-.32	-.22	.16	.18	.05	.11	.11	-.01	.24	1.00				
19.	Close friends	-.06	.08	.01	-.09	-.06	-.07	-.25	.01	.14	.27	-.14	-.20	.21	.09	.08	-.05	.05	.06	1.00			
20.	Age at arrival	.02	.04	-.10	.06	.09	.07	.13	.02	-.23	-.42	.18	.17	-.16	.01	.03	.00	.01	.06	-.12	1.00		
21.	Physical health	-.06	-.05	.05	-.07	.02	-.08	-.07	.02	.10	.31	-.20	-.29	.11	.08	.02	-.02	-.02	.00	.17	-.30	1.00	
22.	Distress (T1)	.36	.12	-.14	.31	.25	.09	.07	.31	-.23	-.17	.37	.14	-.16	-.27	.09	.17	-.05	.03	-.09	.09	-.36	1.00
23.	Distress (T2)	.19	.04	-.07	.20	.17	.03	.17	.17	-.22	-.22	.39	.25	-.19	-.15	-.05	.12	-.08	-.04	-.15	.14	-.31	.43

Source: IHARP Longitudinal Adult Sample, N = 500.

Multiple regression techniques were used to test the general model sketched earlier in Figure 4.1. Table 4.7 presents the results of equations predicting psychological distress at both T1 and T2. Results are given in three columns: first for the adult sample as a whole, and then separately for men and women to test for the possibility that the determination of distress varies by gender. Seven sets of predictor variables were examined for their effects on distress. Each set of predictor variables was entered into the equations in the following order, as shown in Table 4.7: (1) *motives* (type 1, type 2, and type 3 motives); (2) *migration events* (family loss index, traumatic events, and months in camps); (3) *prearrival characteristics* (rural origin, year of arrival); (4) *postarrival socioeconomic adaptation* (labor force participation, income, health care access problems); (5) *cultural adaptation* (attitudinal items measuring assimilationism, biculturalism, traditionalism); (6) *social support* (married or not, number of relatives at home, number of close coethnic friends); and (7) *physical health status* (QWB score). The first three sets involve prearrival factors defining the context of exit, the next three sets are postarrival factors defining the context of entry, and the last is a key covariate (somatic symptoms and dysfunctions). The logic of this order of entry was to examine the effects on distress first of motivational variables (prior to exit), then of migration variables (during exit and prior to arrival), then of adaptation variables (after arrival), and lastly of mediating variables (social support) and health. While the dependent variable (psychological distress) was measured at T1 and T2, almost all of the independent variables used were measured at T1. This permits us to establish unambiguously the causal sequence of effects, and to assess which independent variables increase or decrease in predictive importance over time.

One statistic given in Table 4.7 is the change in the square of the multiple coefficient (ΔR^2). It provides a useful estimate of the net percentage of the "explained" variance contributed by each set of independent variables as it was entered into the equation. To illustrate: at T1, motives explained 15.5 percent of the variance in distress scores (ΔR^2 = .155), migration events contributed another 6.8 percent to the explanation (ΔR^2 = .068), rural origin and year of arrival added 2.5 percent (ΔR^2 = .025), economic adaptation 4.0 percent (ΔR^2 = .040), cultural adaptation 3.3 percent (ΔR^2 = .033), social support only 0.3 percent (ΔR^2 = .003), and finally physical health 7.8 percent (ΔR^2 = .078). Summed together, this model explained a total of 40.2 percent of the variance in psychological distress at T1 (R^2 = .402). Clearly, the prearrival factors explained a great deal more of the refugees' level of distress—24.8 percent (.155 + .068 + .025 = .248)—than did the postarrival factors—only 7.6 percent (.040 + .033 + .003 = .076). A first conclusion, then, is that contexts of exit were about three times more significant than contexts of entry in determining the level of psychological distress experienced by the refugees at T1.

A very different picture emerges from the results a year later at T2, however. Now motives explained only 4.6 percent of the variance in distress scores (R^2 = .046), migration events added only 3.8 percent to the explanation, and rural origin and year of arrival explained only 0.7 percent. By contrast, T2 economic adaptation variables increased significantly in explanatory power to account for 10.3 percent (R^2 = .103), with cultural adaptation (2.3 percent) and social support (0.7 percent) adding modestly to the determination of distress scores. Physical health status contributed another 4.7 percent to the model, bringing the total R^2 to .270 for the overall sample at T2. Thus, the prearrival factors together explained only 9.1 percent of the total variance in T2 distress levels (.046 + .038 + .007 = .091)—a dramatic decrease from their 24.8 percent predictive power at T1—while the postarrival factors doubled their predictive power from 7.6 percent at T1 to 13.3 percent at T2 (.103 + .023 + .007)—a greater proportion of the variance than that accounted for by prearrival factors. The conclusion from these results is inescapable: by T2, contexts of entry had become more important than contexts of exit in shaping the process of psychological adaptation. Past losses and events seem to "heal" with time and recede in importance as present demands and challenges grow in psychological significance. Put another way, over time the "refugees" become more like "immigrants."

A slightly different picture of these processes emerges from the separate regression results for men and women, also displayed in Table 4.7. The patterns of effects change in roughly the same direction for both genders: postarrival factors displace prearrival factors in predictive importance over time. There are some differences worth noting, however. For women, the effects of physical health on mental health are much greater in magnitude than they are for men. For men, by contrast, the effects of migration events and of economic and cultural adaptation on psychological distress are much greater in magnitude than they are for women. There are basically no differences between men and women in the overall magnitude of the psychological effects of motivational factors and social support variables. In general, the regression model explains a greater amount of the total variance in distress scores among men than among women. While these models have substantial explanatory power, it is well to note that much of the variance remains unaccounted for. There are clearly other factors not captured by our data that are involved in the determination of subjective well-being.

So far we have been focusing on the effects of gross sets of predictor

Table 4.7. Predictors of Psychological Distress: Multiple Regression Results for Male and Female Indochinese Refugees at T1 (1983) and T2 (1984)

Analytical Category	Predictor Variables		Total Sample (N = 500)		
			Beta	p^a	ΔR^2
Motives	Motive—type 1	T1	.141	**	
		T2	.054	NS	
	Motive—type 2	T1	.087	*	.155
		T2	.060	NS	.046
	Motive—type 3	T1	−.023	NS	
		T2	−.007	NS	
Migration events	Family loss index	T1	.129	**	
		T2	.056	NS	
	Months in camps	T1	.104	*	.068
		T2	.017	NS	.038
	Migration events	T1	.049	NS	
		T2	.004	NS	
Prearrival characteristics	Year of arrival	T1	−.161	**	.025
		T2	−.035	NS	.007
	Rural origin	T1	.155	**	
		T2	.025	NS	
Postarrival economic adaptation	Access index	T1	.156	**	
		T2	.225	**	
	Not in labor force	T1	.020	NS	.040
		T2	.110	*	.103
	Annual income	T1	−.064	NS	
		T2	−.064	NS	
Cultural adaptation	Accult.—item 1	T1	−.143	**	
		T2	−.109	*	
	Accult.—item 2	T1	.008	NS	.033
		T2	−.136	**	.023
	Accult.—item 3	T1	.094	*	
		T2	.064	NS	
Social support	Married	T1	−.001	NS	
		T2	−.029	NS	
	No. relatives (at home)	T1	−.054	NS	.003
		T2	−.072	NS	.007
	No. close friends (coethnic)	T1	−.002	NS	
		T2	−.050	NS	
Physical health	Physical health (QWB score)	T1	−.310	**	.078
		T2	−.230	**	.047
Total R^2 (explained variance)		T1			.402
		T2			.270

Source: IHARP Longitudinal Adult Sample, N = 500.
Abbreviations: NS, not significant.

Males (N = 248)			Females (N = 252)		
Beta	p	ΔR^2	Beta	p	ΔR^2
.086	NS		.187	**	
.024	NS		.082	NS	
.132	*	.169	.008	NS	.144
.027	NS	.055	.075	NS	.055
.067	NS		−.005	NS	
.038	NS		−.050	NS	
.130	*		.089	NS	
.088	NS		.026	NS	
.078	NS	.096	.080	NS	.051
.015	NS	.069	−.004	NS	.017
.024	NS		.114	*	
−.001	NS		.025	NS	
−.192	**	.018	−.082	NS	.035
−.017	NS	.013	−.021	NS	.002
.114	*		.259	**	
.066	NS		.020	NS	
.182	**		.118	*	
.294	**		.185	**	
.161	**	.085	−.090	NS	.029
.179	**	.139	.039	NS	.065
−.075	NS		−.054	NS	
−.049	NS		−.066	NS	
−.274	**		.025	NS	
−.160	*		−.061	NS	
.072	NS	.066	−.079	NS	.027
−.152	*	.030	−.143	*	.023
.049	NS		.156	**	
−.005	NS		−.111	*	
−.024	NS		−.011	NS	
−.130	*		.058	NS	
.003	NS	.009	−.118	*	.013
.000	NS	.027	−.135	*	.007
−.064	NS		.067	NS	
−.126	*		.009	NS	
−.178	**	.024	−.392	**	.134
−.207	**	.031	−.263	**	.069
		.467			.433
		.364			.237

[a]**$p < .01$; *$p < .05$; NS = not significant; ΔR^2 = change in the R^2 due to *each* of the seven sets of predictor variables.

variables as indicated by the R^2 statistics. A more refined interpretation of these results is possible by examining the standardized regression coefficients (betas) and their level of statistical significance (based on t tests) for each of the independent variables in the model. The betas shown in Table 4.7 are the final coefficients, with all predictor variables entered in the regression equations. That is, they permit a comparison of the relative predictive strength of each variable while controlling for the independent effects of all other variables in the model. To illustrate: at T1, looking first at *motivational factors*, by far the strongest positive predictor of distress are type 1 motives (beta = .141, $p < .01$); type 2 motives exert a weak but still significant positive effect (beta = .087, $p < .05$), while type 3 motives show a negligible though negative association with distress.

Among *migration events*, the strongest determinant of T1 psychological distress is the index of family loss and separation (beta = .129, $p < .01$), followed by months spent in refugee camps overseas (beta = .104, $p < .05$). The global measure of traumatic events experienced in transit, however, is insignificant—for men more so than women. By T2, none of these exit variables retained significant effects on distress levels. Still, underscoring the point made earlier with reference to the literature on unaccompanied children in emergencies, these data suggest that loss and separation from significant objects, rather than the fact of exposure to traumatic flight events, has more impact on the phenomenology of the refugee experience among adults as well. Put another way, distress is decreased when it can be shared. Misery does love company.

Looking at socioeconomic variables in the model, the largest beta coefficients (for both men and women, and at both T1 and T2) were observed for the index of health care access problems: an indicator of powerlessness in one's ability to meet basic needs. For men, being unemployed is strongly and increasingly associated with psychological distress, whereas this effect is not significant for women. Income is revealed not to be a significant predictor of distress once other variables are controlled. Gender differences are also evident with respect to the effects of the various indicators of social support. For men but not for women, being married and having close coethnic friends reduces psychological distress; for women but not for men, having relatives at home serves as a buffer against distress.

It has often been observed that the metaphor of the "melting pot" has never validly characterized American society *as a collectivity*; instead, immigrants have been pressured toward Anglo-conformity as a condition for their acceptance and inclusion (Gordon, 1964). The "melting pot" concept, however, may be more apt as a characterization of the inner agony that immigrants and refugees experience *as individuals* in their adaptation to American life. In this respect, some particularly interesting patterns are observable in Table 4.7 with respect to acculturative attitudes. For men but not for women, acculturation item 1 measuring *assimilationism* is significantly and negatively associated with distress, suggesting that a more open and accommodative attitude toward cultural adaptation reduces symptoms of anxiety and depression. The magnitude of the beta coefficient for this effect among men had been nearly halved by T2, however, though it remained significant. For women but not for men, item 3 measuring *traditionalism* is significantly and positively associated with distress, pointing to the distressing effects of cultural alienation and shock. These contrasting patterns reflect the fact that Indochinese refugee women are more socially isolated than men in America. But for both men and women, and perhaps of greatest interest, is the finding that acculturation item 2 measuring *biculturalism*, which showed insignificant effects on distress at T1, had emerged as a strong negative predictor of distress by T2. That is, refugees who adopt an innovative bicultural strategy toward adaptation significantly reduce their level of psychological distress over time. This finding points to the importance of creativity and flexibility in the acculturative process. It appears that the most successful psychological adjustment is made not by those who remain unacculturated and alienated from the American milieu, nor by those who pursue a monocultural assimilative strategy, but by those who are oriented toward an additive style of acculturation, adapting to American ways while retaining their ethnic identity and attachments.

THE CHILDREN

The SARYS Study: Sample and Sources of Data

During 1986–1987 we conducted a follow-up study on the adaptation of Indochinese children—the Southeast Asian Refugee Youth Study (SARYS). From the IHARP T1 random sample of refugee parents (including the Lao) we identified all their school-age children enrolled in the San Diego (California) Unified School District. Complete academic histories for this sample of Indochinese students [including grade point averages (GPAs) and standardized achievement test scores] were then obtained from the school district and matched with our data on their parents and households, producing an exceptionally in-depth data base. Combined IHARP-school district data were thus collected on 340 elementary school children (kindergarten through grade 6) and on 239 secondary school students (grades 7 through 12). Additional information was collected on school suspensions and dropout rates, and (for high school students) on their occupational aspirations. (For additional details and results of the SARYS study, see Rumbaut and Ima, 1988.)

We turn now to an analysis of characteristics and determinants of their educational attainment, focusing on the subsample of 239 Indochinese secondary school students. By definition, this subsample is representative only of children who came accompanied by one or both parents; it does not include the relatively small minority of children who came without their parents, nor does it include second-generation children who have been born in the United States. Rather, they are members of what we earlier called the "1.5" generation of refugee youth who were born in Southeast Asia but are being educated and coming of age in America. Moreover, the characteristics of the parents of this student subsample are not representative of the larger universe of refugee adults, since childless couples, single or elderly adults, and parents whose children are not enrolled in San Diego city schools are excluded by definition. About half of the adults in the T1 IHARP sample had school-age children meeting our criteria for inclusion in the SARYS student subsample. Still, as will be seen below, the socioeconomic profile of the refugee households in the SARYS study matches in most essential respects that of the groups in the larger IHARP study reviewed above.

Characteristics of Indochinese Refugee Children in Secondary Schools

Table 4.8 presents relevant data for each of the five main ethnic groups (Vietnamese, Chinese-Vietnamese, Hmong, Khmer, and Lao) in the secondary school student subsample. Among them, Vietnamese and Chinese students show the highest levels of educational attainment: they have higher academic GPAs and higher standardized test scores in math and reading achievement. Less than half of the Vietnamese and Chinese are classified by the school district as Limited-English-Proficient (LEP); the majority are classified as Fluent-English-Proficient (FEP). Although their reading scores are below the national average, reflecting their limitations with the English language as recently arrived newcomers, their GPAs are well above those for white Anglos (U.S.-born English-monolingual, white majority students of European ancestry) in the district (and for that matter, all other native-born students) and their math achievement scores place them in the top quartile of the nation—a striking and remarkable level of performance. Cambodian and Lao students, on the other hand, show the lowest levels of attainment both in GPAs and test scores among the refugee groups. Nevertheless, their GPAs match the white Anglo norm and their math scores are at about the national average. So far the ranking of these four groups exactly parallels that of their parents' education: that is, Vietnamese parents

Table 4.8. Academic Grade Point Averages, Standardized Achievement Test Scores, and Characteristics of Indochinese Refugee Students and Their Families, by Ethnic Group

Characteristics	Vietnamese (N = 54)	Chinese (N = 45)	Khmer (N = 35)	Lao (N = 58)	Hmong (N = 47)	p^a	Total (N = 239)
Educational Attainment							
Academic grade point average[b]	2.97	2.88	2.64	2.57	2.78	*	2.77
CTBS reading test score[c]	4.07	3.45	3.30	2.78	2.96	**	3.34
CTBS math test score[c]	6.97	6.80	4.81	5.48	5.73	**	6.09
% Limited English status (LEP)[d]	48.1	42.2	74.3	77.6	55.3	**	59.4
Family situation							
% Live in two-parent household	90.7	91.1	45.7	82.8	83.0	**	89.7
% Below poverty line	61.1	77.8	73.5	82.8	80.9	**	75.2
Parents' characteristics							
Parents' education (years)	8.9	5.7	4.4	3.8	1.3	**	4.9
Mother's English literacy	1.85	1.00	1.15	1.05	1.10	**	1.25
Parents' acculturation attitudes	3.54	4.14	4.03	3.99	4.24	**	3.97
Mother's psychological distress	1.57	1.37	2.14	1.75	1.70	**	1.69
Students' characteristics							
Year born in S.E. Asia (19___)	70.3	70.0	69.3	70.0	69.6	NS	69.9
Year arrived in United States (19___)	78.3	79.9	80.1	79.6	79.1	**	79.3
Semesters in U.S. secondary schools	5.0	5.4	4.2	4.4	5.2	*	4.9
% Male students	51.8	51.1	51.4	44.8	57.4	NS	51.0

Source: IHARP Subsample, N = 239 students, grades 7–12.

Abbreviations: NS, not significant.

[a]Significance (p) of differences between ethnic groups: **$p < .01$, *$p < .05$.

[b]Cumulative academic grade point average, excluding physical education courses, where: A = 4, B = 3, C = 2, D = 1, F = 0.

[c]Scores achieved on the reading (English vocabulary and comprehension) and math subtests of the CTBS (Comprehensive Test of Basic Skills), a nationally standardized achievement test given annually to all students in San Diego City Schools and widely used by schools throughout the United States. Results in the table are presented in STANINE scores: a standardized scale of nine units, scored 1 (low)–9 (high), distributed normally (a bell-shaped curve) with a mean of 5 and a standard deviation of 2. A score of 1 thus places students in the bottom 4% nationally and a score of 9 in the top 4% nationally, while a score of 5 places students in the middle 20% nationally among same-grade-level peers who took the CTBS.

[d]Schools classify students whose primary language at home is not English (as is the case for all Indochinese students) as either LEP (limited-English-proficient) or FEP (fluent-English-proficient). A FEP classification implies a minimum level of English competence sufficient to justify mainstreaming the student from ESL (English as a Second Language) to regular courses.

are the most educated, followed by Chinese, Cambodians, and Lao. What is surprising is that Hmong occupy an intermediate position in both GPAs and test scores between these four other groups—despite the fact that Hmong parents have by far the least amount of education (averaging just above the first grade level). Thus, the refugee students' current educational achievement is not simply a function of their parents' social class of origin.

About 75 percent of all of these students live in households with incomes below the federal poverty line; their families are among the poorest in the San Diego area. About 90 percent of the Vietnamese and Chinese live in intact homes with both parents, as do about 83 percent of the Hmong and the Lao. But less than half of the Cambodians live in two-parent households; most live with widowed mothers, again reflecting the extremely high death rates in Cambodia during the Pol Pot period of the late 1970s. Cambodian mothers also show the most elevated levels of depressive symptomatology, followed by Hmong and Lao mothers, with the Vietnamese and Chinese reflecting the best mental health profiles. The bottom panel of Table 4.8 provides information on basic student characteristics: there are no significant differences in age or gender among the students in the sample, but the Cambodians and the Lao are the most recently arrived groups and hence have fewer semesters in U.S. secondary schools and a higher proportion of LEP students. Time is clearly a key variable shaping the adaptation process of these groups, along with parental socioeconomic and psychocultural factors.

Determinants of Educational Achievement

All of these independent variables (as well as many others not shown here) were examined for their effects on two key indicators of educational attainment: GPAs and English reading achievement test scores. The results of a multiple regression analysis are presented in Table 4.9. Because of multicollinearity between the two variables of parents' education and level of English literacy ($r = .70$), a single index was produced by summing both of these indicators of parental social class resources. The method followed in the analysis is similar to that used above. In each regression analysis three sets of predictor variables were entered into the equation one at a time: (1) first, a set of *ethnicity* dummy variables were entered (with the Chinese as the reference group); (2) next a set of *family* characteristics were entered, for the purpose of assessing the effects of parental composition and social class, as well as cultural and psychological variables that are not often considered in analyses of educational attainment; and lastly (3) a set of *student* char-

Table 4.9. Predictors of English Reading Achievement Test Scores (Y_1) and Academic GPA (Y_2) Among Indochinese Refugee Students in San Diego City Schools: Results of Multiple Regression Analyses for Sample of Secondary School Children[a]

Analytical Category	Predictor Variables (X_n)	$Y_1 = $ Reading Score			$Y_2 = $ GPA		
		Beta	p	ΔR^2	Beta	p	ΔR^2
Ethnicity	Vietnamese (Yes = 1, No = 0)	.079	NS		.216	**	
	Cambodian (Yes = 1, No = 0)	−0.10	NS		.135	NS	
	Hmong (Yes = 1, No = 0)	−.097	NS	.101	.073	NS	.035
	Lao (Yes = 1, No = 0)	−.092	NS		.040	NS	
Parents' characteristics	Parents' education + English literacy	.153	*		.001	NS	
	Two-parent home (Yes = 1, No = 0)	−.101	NS		−.024	NS	
	Below poverty (Yes = 1, No = 0)	−.067	NS	.178	−.076	NS	.120
	Parents' acculturation attitudes	.105	NS		.245	**	
	Psychological distress (mother)	−.029	NS		−.176	**	
Students' characteristics	Year born (19__)	.277	**		.448	**	
	Year of arrival in United States (19__)	−.277	**		.157	*	
	Semesters (in U.S. secondary schools)	.042	NS	.194	.359	**	.177
	English status (FEP = 1, LEP = 0)	.262	**		.264	**	
	Gender (male = 1, female = 0)	−.030	NS		−.074	NS	
Total R^2 (explained variance) =				.473			.332

Source: IHARP subsample, $N = 239$ students, grades 7–12.
Abbreviations: FEP, fluent-English-proficient; LEP, limited-English-proficient; NS, not significant.
[a]Significance levels for betas: **$p < .01$; *$p < .05$. The betas shown are the final standardized regression coefficients with all variables entered in the equation. R^2 = square of total multiple correlation for each equation. ΔR^2 = change in the R^2 (or explained variance) due to *each* of the three sets of predictor variables as each set was entered into the equation (ethnicity variables were entered first, then parents' characteristics, and finally students' characteristics).

acteristics to control for age, sex, FEP or LEP status, time in the United States, and semesters in U.S. secondary schools. The change in the square of the multiple correlation (ΔR^2)—that is, the percent of the variance accounted for by each set of predictors as it was entered into the equation—is noted in Table 4.9 at each step, and the total R^2 for each model is given at the bottom of the table. The final betas or standardized regression coefficients in the equations are also noted for each predictor variable, with all other variables controlled.

Turning to the results on English reading achievement, the regression model accounted for nearly half of the variance in test scores ($R^2 = .473$). The set of ethnicity variables, entered first, accounted for 10.1 percent of the variance; however, the betas for the specific ethnic variables were not significant when other variables were controlled. The set of parental characteristics contributed another 17.8 percent to the explanation of English reading test scores; the key predictor variable here was the parents' level of education and English literacy (beta = .153, $p <$ .05). None of the other parental and family variables had a significant effect on these test scores. Finally, the set of students' characteristics added another 19.4 percent to the explanatory power of the model. Reading scores were not significantly different by gender. With FEP and LEP status controlled, the strongest predictor variables were the students' age and time in the United States (as opposed to semesters in school): that is, the younger the students and the longer in the United States, the better their reading ability in English. Interestingly, this finding parallels our analysis of adults' level of English literacy in the larger IHARP sample: the main predictors were their level of premigration education, (younger) age at arrival, and amount of time in the United States (Rumbaut, R. G., 1989a). While this is a parsimonious model with considerable explanatory power, more than half of the variance in reading scores remains unexplained by the predictor variables in the model. Clearly other causal dynamics are at work that are not encompassed by the variables tested here.

Turning next to the analysis of GPAs, the regression model accounted for 33 percent of the variance (R^2 = .332). Ethnicity alone accounted for just 3.5 percent of the variance in GPAs. However, with all variables controlled, Vietnamese ethnicity emerged as a strong positive predictor of GPAs, underscoring the fact that Vietnamese students had the highest GPAs in the school district. The set of student characteristics contributed 17.7 percent to the explanation of GPAs. All of these variables except gender showed significant positive effects: the younger the students and the longer in U.S. schools (where they "learn the ropes" of the American school system), the higher their GPA; and FEP students (fluent bilinguals) clearly had an advantage over those classified as LEP (limited bilinguals). The set of parental and family characteristics explained another 12 percent of the variance in GPAs. But notably, the significant predictors of GPA here were not the more "objective" variables measuring parental education or poverty or family composition, but rather two "subjective" psychocultural variables: (1) the more *psychologically distressed* the mother, the lower the student's GPA—a finding that underscores the pivotal role of mothers in their children's upbringing, and shows that psychological distress among refugee adults is a significant causal variable in its own right affecting the adaptation of their children; and (2) the greater the parents' score on an index of *acculturation attitudes*, the higher the GPA.

The parents' acculturation score is a summed index of four items, each item measured on a 0 to 6 scale from "strongly disagree" to "strongly agree," with 3 as a neutral midpoint. (The items were drawn from the same set of attitudinal items we reported above in the analysis of the adult cultural adaptation process; the first of these is the item we earlier termed *biculturalism.*) Specifically, the four items expressed the degree to which refugee parents felt that (1) their ethnic group must stay together as a community to preserve their own culture and identity even as they adapt to the American economy to "make a living"; (2) they should stick together as a group for social support and mutual assistance; (3) they should live in coethnic neighborhoods; and (4) they would *not* return to their homelands even if there were a change in government. This index thus provides a general measure not of assimilation or "Americanization," but rather of a sense of ethnic resilience and solidarity among parents who intend to stay in the United States and to do so while affirming their ethnic culture and social networks. The higher this score, the higher the GPA of their children. This finding runs counter to assimilationist assumptions that argue that the more acculturated and Americanized immigrants become, the greater will be their success in the competitive worlds of school and work. In fact, it suggests an opposite conclusion: namely, that "Americanization" processes may be dysfunctional for educational attainment.

In summary, then, we found that parental socioeconomic status is more predictive of reading test scores than of GPA. That is, objective family characteristics did not affect GPA directly, a result that suggests that their influence is mediated by other factors, such as knowledge of English. By contrast, the set of more subjective variables—the parents' "psychocultural status"—is strongly predictive of GPA, but not of test scores. This finding points to the importance for GPA of cultural, attitudinal, and emotional factors in parent-child (and especially mother-child) relationships, with GPA seen here as a measure of attainment based to a considerable extent on "motivated effort" rather than simply on "talent" or "luck." Of these, of greater import is the parents' affirmation of ethnic identity and solidarity within family and community structures. Finally, age and time variables are important. The (younger) age of the student is predictive of higher GPAs and test scores. But time in the United States has a different effect—and meaning—depending on age at arrival. Based on our ethnographic work (Rumbaut and Ima, 1988), the key difference involves those youth whose age at arrival in the United States was prepuberty (or roughly younger than 12 years) versus those who arrived postpuberty in their later teens. The older students are more handicapped by language deficiencies, may have "lost" more time from normal schooling during their often-prolonged stays in refugee camps overseas, may have had less time to learn the ropes of the new system, and must cope simultaneously with the additional developmental stressors of middle and late adolescence.

We believe, however, that the finding that educational achievement improves for younger refugees and over time in the United States cannot be projected indefinitely. Rather, we predict that this effect will soon plateau and then begin to diminish if and when the younger family members become more inculcated with values prevailing among American youth which (according to national poll data) emphasize self-fulfillment and gratification over self-sacrifice and hard work—a process of "becoming American" that may ironically prove counterproductive for educational attainment in competitive school settings. Younger refugees, even though their English competency and their knowledge of American society is better, may become less driven and less single-minded in their pursuit of school and work goals, and thus at some point less apt to reach the levels of attainment achieved by their more motivated and harder-working older siblings. The exact level of educational and work achievement during the transition to living in American society will depend on the ability of Southeast Asian families to develop and maintain bicultural values, norms, and pressures that lead to high achievement regardless of the social class resources of the parents, and that assist both parents and children in bridging effectively their native and adoptive worlds. In their own way and not without cost, Indochinese refugee youth are engaged in a process of constructing a world of choice and not of fate. For all of them, the process will be a lifetime occupation.

REFERENCES

Antonovsky, A. (1979). *Health, Stress, and Coping*. San Francisco: Jossey-Bass.

Antonovsky, A. (1987). *Unraveling the Mystery of Health: How People Manage Stress and Stay Well*. San Francisco: Jossey-Bass.

Baskauskas, L. (1981). The Lithuanian refugee experience and grief. *International Migration Review, 15*(1–2), 276–291.

Beiser, M. (1987). Changing time perspective and mental health among Southeast Asian refugees. *Culture, Medicine, and Psychiatry, 11*, 437–464.

Beiser, M. (1988). Influences of time, ethnicity, and attachment on depression in Southeast Asian refugees. *American Journal of Psychiatry, 145*(1), 46–51.

Berry, J. W. (1986). The acculturation process and refugee behavior. In C. L. Williams and J. Westermeyer (eds.), *Refugee Mental Health in Resettlement Countries*, pp. 25–37. New York: Hemisphere.

Berry, J. W., Uichol, K., Minde, T., and Mok, D. (1987). Comparative studies of acculturative stress. *International Migration Review, 21*(3), 491–511.

Carlin, J. E. (1979). The catastrophically uprooted child: Southeast Asian refugee children. In J. D. Call, J. D. Noshpitz, R. L. Cohen, and I. N. Berlin (eds.), *Basic Handbook of Childhood Psychiatry*, Vol. 1, pp. 290–300. New York: Basic Books.

Carlin, J. E. (1986). Child and adolescent refugees: Psychiatric assessment and treatment. In C. L. Williams and J. Westermeyer (eds.), *Refugee Mental Health in Resettlement Countries*, pp. 131–139. New York: Hemisphere.

Chan, K. B., and Loveridge, D. (1987). Refugees "in transit": Vietnamese in a refugee camp in Hong Kong. *International Migration Review, 21*(3), 745–759.

Cohon, J. D. (1981). Psychological adaptation and dysfunction among refugees. *International Migration Review, 15*(1–2), 255–275.

David, H. P. (1970). Involuntary international migration: Adaptation of refugees. In E. B. Brody (ed.), *Behavior in New Environments: Adaptation of Migrant Populations*, pp. 73–95. Beverly Hill, Calif.: Sage.

Furnham, A., and Bochner, S. (1986). *Culture Shock: Psychological Reactions to Unfamiliar Environments*. New York: Methuen.

Garza-Guerrero, A. C. (1974). Culture shock: Its mourning and the vicissitudes of identity. *Journal of the American Psychoanalytic Association, 22*, 408–429.

Gordon, M. M. (1964). *Assimilation in American Life*. New York: Oxford University Press.

Haines, D. W. (ed.) (1985). *Refugees in the United States: A Reference Handbook*. Westport, Conn.: Greenwood.

Isaacs, A. R. (1983). *Without Honor: Defeat in Vietnam and Cambodia*. Baltimore: Johns Hopkins University Press.

Karnow, S. (1983). *Vietnam: A History*. New York: Viking Press.

Kinzie, J. D., Sack, W. H., Angell, R., Manson, S., and Rath, B. (1986). The psychiatric effects of massive trauma on Cambodian children. *Journal of the American Academy of Child Psychiatry, 25*, 370–376.

Knudsen, J. C. (1983). *Boat People in Transit: Vietnamese in Refugee Camps in the Philippines, Hong Kong and Japan*. Series in Social Anthropology, No. 31. Bergen, Norway: University of Bergen.

Kunz, E. F. (1973). The refugee in flight: Kinetic models and forms of displacement. *International Migration Review, 7*(2), 125–146.

Kunz, E. F. (1981). Exile and resettlement: Refugee theory. *International Migration Review, 15*(1–2), 42–51.

Lin, K.-M. (1986). Psychopathology and social disruption in refugees. In C. L. Williams and J. Westermeyer (eds.), *Refugee Mental Health in Resettlement Countries*, pp. 61–73. New York: Hemisphere.

Lin, K.-M., Tazuma, L., and Masuda, M. (1979). Adaptational problems of Vietnamese refugees: I. Health and mental health status. *Archives of General Psychiatry, 36*, 955–961.

Link, B., and Dohrenwend, B. P. (1980). Formulation of hypotheses about the true prevalence of demoralization. In B. P. Dohrenwend (ed.), *Mental Illness in the United States: Epidemiological Estimates*, pp. 114–132. New York: Praeger.

Liu, W. T., Lamanna, M., and Murata, A. (1979). *Transition to Nowhere: Vietnamese Refugees in America*. Nashville, Tenn.: Charter House.

Mason, L., and Brown, R. (1983). *Rice, Rivalry, and Politics: Managing Cambodian Relief*. Notre Dame, Ind.: University of Notre Dame Press.

Masuda, M., Lin, K.-M., and Tazuma, L. (1980). Adaptational problems of Vietnamese refugees: II. Life changes and perceptions of life events. *Archives of General Psychiatry, 37*, 447–450.

Meinhardt, K., Tom, S., Tse, P., and Yu, C. Y. (1985–1986). Southeast Asian refugees in the "Silicon Valley": The Asian Health Assessment Project. *Amerasia, 12*(2), 43–65.

Milburn, T. W., and Watman, K. H. (1981). *On the Nature of Threat: A Social Psychological Analysis.* New York: Praeger.

Mirowsky, J., and Ross, C. E. (1986). Social patterns of distress. *Annual Review of Sociology, 12*, 23–45.

Mollica, R. F., and Lavelle, J. P. (1988). Southeast Asian refugees. In L. Comas-Díaz and E.E.H. Griffith (eds.), *Clinical Guidelines in Cross-Cultural Mental Health*, pp. 262–302. New York: Wiley.

Oberg, K. (1960). Cultural shock: Adjustment to new cultural environments. *Practical Anthropology, 7*, 177–182.

Owan, T. C. (ed.) (1985). *Southeast Asian Mental Health: Treatment, Prevention, Services, Training, and Research.* Rockville, Md.: National Institute of Mental Health.

Pedraza-Bailey, S. (1985). *Political and Economic Migrants in America.* Austin: University of Texas Press.

Portes, A., and Rumbaut, R. G. (1990). *Immigrant America: A Portrait.* Berkeley: University of California Press.

Ressler, E. M., Boothby, N., and Steinbock, D. J. (1988). *Unaccompanied Children: Care and Protection in Wars, Natural Disasters, and Refugee Movements.* New York: Oxford University Press.

Rose, P. I. (1981). Some thoughts about refugees and the descendants of Theseus. *International Migration Review, 15*(1–2), 8–15.

Rosenblatt, R. (1984). *Children of War.* Garden City, N.Y.: Doubleday.

Rumbaut, R. D. (1977). Life events, change, migration, and depression. In W. E. Fann, I. Karacan, A. D. Pokorny, and R. L. Williams (eds.), *Phenomenology and Treatment of Depression*, pp. 115–126. New York: Plenum.

Rumbaut, R. D., and Rumbaut, R. G. (1976). The family in exile: Cuban expatriates in the United States. *American Journal of Psychiatry, 133*(4), 395–399.

Rumbaut, R. G. (1976). Two generational perspectives on the experience of exile: Crisis, commitment, and identity. Presented at the Annual Meeting of the American Society for Adolescent Psychiatry, Miami, Fla.

Rumbaut, R. G. (1985). Mental health and the refugee experience: A comparative study of Southeast Asian refugees. In T. C. Owan (ed.), *Southeast Asian Mental Health*, pp. 433–486. Rockville, Md.: National Institute of Mental Health.

Rumbaut, R. G. (1989a). Portraits, patterns and predictors of the refugee adaptation process. In D. W. Haines (ed.), *Refugees as Immigrants: Cambodians, Laotians, and Vietnamese in America*, pp. 138–182. Totowa, N.J.: Rowman & Littlefield.

Rumbaut, R. G. (1989b). The structure of refuge: Southeast Asian refugees in the United States, 1975–1985. *International Review of Comparative Public Policy*, 1, 97–129.

Rumbaut, R. G., Chávez, L. R., Moser, R. J., Pickwell, S. M., and Wishik, S. M. (1988). The politics of migrant health care: A comparative study of Mexican immigrants and Indochinese refugees. *Research in the Sociology of Health Care*, 7, 143–202.

Rumbaut, R. G., and Ima, K. (1988). *The Adaptation of Southeast Asian Refugee Youth: A Comparative Study.* Washington, D.C.: U.S. Office of Refugee Resettlement.

Rumbaut, R. G., and Weeks, J. R. (1986). Fertility and adaptation: Indochinese refugees in the United States. *International Migration Review*, 20(2), 428–466.

Shawcross, W. (1984). *The Quality of Mercy: Cambodia, Holocaust and Modern Conscience.* New York: Simon and Schuster.

Stein, B. N. (1986). The experience of being a refugee: Insights from the research literature. In C. L. Williams and J. Westermeyer (eds.), *Refugee Mental Health in Resettlement Countries*, pp. 5–23. New York: Hemisphere.

Stonequist, E. V. (1937). *The Marginal Man: A Study in Personality and Culture Conflict.* New York: Russell & Russell.

Strand, P. J., and Jones, W., Jr. (1985). *Indochinese Refugees in America.* Durham, N.C.: Duke University Press.

Tobin, J. J., and Friedman, J. (1984). Intercultural and developmental stresses confronting Southeast Asian refugee adolescents. *Journal of Operational Psychiatry*, 15, 39–45.

Tyhurst, L. (1951). Displacement and migration: A study in social psychiatry. *American Journal of Psychiatry*, 101, 561–568.

Tyhurst, L. (1977). Psychosocial first aid for refugees: An essay in social psychiatry. *Mental Health and Society*, 4, 319–343.

U.S. Committee for Refugees (1984). *Vietnamese Boat People: Pirates' Vulnerable Prey.* Washington, D.C.: Author.

U.S. Committee for Refugees (1985). *Cambodians in Thailand: People on the Edge.* Washington, D.C.: Author.

U.S. Committee for Refugees (1986). *Refugees from Laos: In Harm's Way.* Washington, D.C.: Author.

U.S. Committee for Refugees (1988). *Refugee Reports*, 9(12), 1–15.

U.S. Committee for Refugees (1989). *World Refugee Survey—1988 in Review.* Washington, D.C.: American Council for Nationalities Service.

Williams, C. L., and Westermeyer, J. (eds.) (1986). *Refugee Mental Health in Resettlement Countries.* New York: Hemisphere.

5 Severely Traumatized Cambodian Children: Research Findings and Clinical Implications

J. DAVID KINZIE, M.D., and WILLIAM SACK, M.D.

Until 1970, Cambodia was a relatively rich Southeast Asian country with ample natural resources and a productive agriculture. Most Cambodians lived in small villages near waterways, and the majority of the people were engaged in agriculture. Traditionally, Buddhist monks and high government officials received high social status, but high status was also given to those with educational, political, or economic success.

Traditional values included a strong family identity, a respect for family ancestors and the past, and a need to maintain smooth personal relationships. Both Hindu and Buddhist religions influenced these values, although the predominant faith was Buddhism. Cambodians believed in reincarnation and that their current life successes or failures depended upon events in a previous life. Along with Buddhism was a strong folk belief in spirits and supernatural influence affecting events.

The Indochinese War expanded into Cambodia in 1970, when the Lon Nol government replaced Prince Sihanouk. In mid-1975, the Communist government of the Pol Pot Khmer Rouge gained control of Cambodia. The deaths and destruction that followed under this regime have been detailed in recent books (Ablin and Hood, 1987; Becker, 1986). Between one and three million of the seven million Cambodian population died under this regime. Hundreds of thousands were executed. Others died of starvation and disease brought about by forced urban evacuation and brutal labor camps.

Particularly singled out for execution were Buddhist monks, urban dwellers, and those with a Western education. In the labor camps, husbands were separated from wives, and children above the age of 6 usually were put in age-related camps away from their families. The regime struck at the fabric of traditional Cambodian life by destroying contact with the past, the religion, the educational system, and the family. This destruction has been called "autogenicide" (Hawk, 1982)—atrocities perpetuated by Cambodians on Cambodians.

Since 1978, the Department of Psychiatry of Oregon Health Sciences University has maintained a clinic for Indochinese refugees. In the early 1980s, some of the Cambodians who had been through Pol Pot and were refugees in Thailand began to come to the United States. Slowly we recognized that the effects of massive trauma endured by these people resulted in different clinical presentations from those of other refugees. We identified post-traumatic stress disorder (PTSD) among Cambodians (Kinzie et al., 1984) as described in *Diagnostic and Statistical Manual of Mental Disorders,* 3rd ed. (*DSM-III*) and subsequently in *Diagnostic and Statistical Manual of Mental Disorders,* 3rd ed. revised (*DSM-IIIR*).

Further work over the next six years indicated that the disorder was common among Cambodians seen in a psychiatric clinic and that the syndrome tended to run a chronic course (Boehnlein et al., 1985; Kinzie, 1986). Many intrusive symptoms seemed to improve with time, particularly nightmares, sleep disorders, and intrusive thoughts. However, the avoidance symptoms (avoiding thoughts and feelings associated with the trauma, psychogenic amnesia, and feelings of detachment) did not improve. All patients remaind extremely vulnerable to stress and under even minimal stress had a full activation of the syndrome.

STUDY OF FORTY CAMBODIAN STUDENTS TRAUMATIZED AS CHILDREN IN CAMBODIA

In the mid-1980s, the authors were approached by the staff of a Portland high school to help them understand some of the behaviors exhibited by their Cambodian students. Teachers had observed clear examples of students showing sudden fear reactions or reexperiencing phenomena to stimuli in the classroom. With the cooperation of school officials and families, we performed semistructured psychiatric interviews with 46 of the 52 Cambodian students in the school (Kinzie et al., 1986; Sack et al., 1986).

The standardized interview included a major portion of the Schedule for Affective Disorders and Schizophrenia (SADS) (Spitzer and Endicott, 1979) as well as structured questions on PTSD taken from the Diagnostic Instrument Schedule (DIS) (Robins et al., 1982). Mental status examination questions were included and any ambiguities or nonverbal reactions were noted during the interview. Three psychiatrists did all the interviews and were aided by the same Cambodian mental health worker, who had six years' experience in interpretation and mental health counseling in an American clinic.

Six of the 46 students had left Cambodia before Pol Pot and therefore suffered no major traumas and had no major symptoms. The remaining 40 students (25 boys, 15 girls), with an average age of 17 (ages 14 to 20), were included in the first study (T1). Generally they had had about eight years of normal Cambodian life before their four years in Pol Pot concentration camps. They averaged two years of school before Pol Pot, although some had further education as refugees in Thailand. All had massive trauma. Thirty-six lived in age-related camps; almost all endured forced labor, often 15 hours a day, seven days a week; 33 went without adequate food for long periods of time; and 27 starved, describing themselves as "looking like a skeleton." Seventeen students saw people killed and seven saw their own family members killed. The number of lost family members, that is, killed or missing, was extremely high: 32 of the 40 students lost at least one family member; the net average number either dead or missing from their nuclear family was three.

Psychiatric disorders were very common. Twenty (50 percent) suffered PTSD by *DSM-III* standards (19 by *DSM-IIIR*). Depressive disorders were present in 21 (53 percent), but 15 of these were intermittent disorders of a mild type. Panic disorders and generalized anxiety were also present and 27 had at least one Axis I diagnosis. Surprisingly, there were no cases of drug or alcohol abuse, and no antisocial or conduct disorders. Not all of the children had a diagnosis but those who did had a much lower Children's Global Assessment Score (CGAS) (Shaffer et al., 1983) than those without a diagnosis.

There was no relationship between age, sex, or experiences in Cambodia and the presence of a diagnosis. There was no simple direct relationship between a specific reported experience (seeing the death of a family member, seeing people being beaten, going without food, suffering severe starvation) and a PTSD or other diagnosis or a CGAS. There was a strong relationship between the current living situation and the psychiatric diagnosis. Twenty-six of the 40 students lived with one or more nuclear family members, while 14 lived in a Cambodian or American foster home. Thirteen of 14 living in foster homes received psychiatric diagnoses, while only 14 of the 26 living with a nuclear family member received such diagnoses. It was our impression that those having reestablished some contact with family members mitigated some of the symptoms of severe trauma, while being alone or in a foster home exacerbated such symptoms. We were also impressed by the lack of social impairment and antisocial behavior in this group. We thought that the continued presence of traditional Cambodian and Buddhist values instilled in the first eight years of family life prevented antisocial activity despite the occurrence of other symptoms.

We sought more information about the students by means of home interviews and teachers' ratings. We found that the students reported more distress with their grades and peer relationships than any reported or observed by their caretakers, that is, teachers or parents. It also became apparent during home interviews that many of the family members exhibited similar post-traumatic stress or depressive symptoms. Those students who received psychiatric diagnoses were usually rated by their classroom teachers as withdrawn or daydreamers but not as disruptive or suffering from any conduct disorder. The school seemed to be a critical culture element in maintaining these students during this difficult adjustment period as refugees and victims of severe trauma.

THREE-YEAR FOLLOW-UP OF TRAUMATIZED CAMBODIAN CHILDREN

A follow-up study gives a valuable history and prognosis of disorders. This is especially important when evaluating children who suffer from massive psychological trauma since few relevant studies are available. Because the Cambodian children were studied previously and had had a protective school environment, it was important to see how adult life and facing the stressors of working, marriage, and of moving away from home affected their symptoms and disorders.

Three years after the original study, we began a follow-up study on these Cambodian young people (Kinzie et al., 1989). The psychiatrists and mental health worker involved were the same as in the first interview and the methodology was the same, with the addition of questions about the students' current adjustment through the use of the Social Adjustment Scale (SAS) (Weissman et al., 1981) and the use of two self-rating scales, the Beck Depression Inventory (Beck et al., 1961) and the Impact of Events Scale (Zilberg et al., 1982).

Before we proceed, a word of caution about the instruments is in order. None of the instruments we used have been normed on Cambodian populations, thus we have no cross-cultural psychometric data. We are currently conducting studies on the factor structure of the Beck Depression Inventory in Cambodian populations, and are doing test and retest reliability studies on the Beck Depression Inventory, the Impact of Events Scale, and the Kiddic Schedule for Affective Disorder and Schizophrenia (K-SADS) on a group of Cambodian adolescents. We do feel the data obtained has strong face validity since the data square with our clinical experience.

We were able to interview 27 of the original 40 students even though some resided as far away as California and Massachusetts. At follow-up (T2), almost all were living with Cambodians, having moved out of

American foster homes. Fifteen of these students were still in school and 15 were supporting themselves, but 60 percent were on welfare.

During the follow-up period, four of the original subjects had received some therapy (it was offered to all who were in distress at the first interview) and one was currently in therapy. At follow-up, 13 individuals (48 percent) had PTSD and 11 had some depressive disorder. The depressive disorder now tended to be more major than minor or intermittent and was associated with PTSD. Panic and anxiety disorders had diminished greatly but one person developed alcohol abuse. There was no diagnosis of schizophrenia, and no antisocial behavior was reported.

Subjects with PTSD tended to be more impaired than those without, although specific items of work and of social and family relations on the SAS did not show a difference. Indeed, most of the Cambodian subjects seemed to be doing reasonably well. The major problems seemed to be related to PTSD. Those with PTSD tended to have higher Beck Depression Inventory scores, and both those with and without PTSD tended to have high avoidance behavior regarding trauma reported on the Impact of Events Scale. Clearly the presence of PTSD was the most significant finding in the follow-up; other symptoms had waned somewhat. PTSD with nightmares, intrusive thoughts, avoidance behavior, and symptoms of arousal continued to be present over eight years after the ending of the trauma in Cambodia.

Interestingly, PTSD tended to remain stable for some of the students. Eleven individuals had PTSD both times (T1 and T2), but it was not apparent at either time in 13. There were three subjects whose PTSD diminished over the three years, but five showed PTSD for the first time at T2. Thus, there remained a group of eight subjects for which PTSD symptoms fluctuated over time. Although suffering and symptoms were present in all at follow-up, there were no conduct disturbances or antisocial acts; mainly the patients' suffering was subjective and private.

CASE HISTORIES

The following Cambodian young people had complicated and variable histories, not only of the trauma they endured but their reaction to it. The research data failed to describe adequately the tremendous stresses they endured or the variety of responses and adjustments to stress. Their case histories provide only a glimpse of their difficulties and their reactions to them.

Case 1: As a preteenager, M. lived in a small city in Cambodia where he attended school for two years. He remembered his life was happy; his father provided for the family well through his trading business. When Pol Pot came to power, a sister and her husband were killed, and the father developed a high fever and died. M.'s mother had a miscarriage and died about one month later. There was a forced separation and M. never again heard of any of his three younger sisters and an older brother. He denied seeing any killings but did see "corpses all over the place." He did forced labor from eight in the morning until six at night every day, working on dikes and growing rice. He went for long periods without food and lost much weight, but denied any specific injuries. He escaped from Cambodia in 1979 when he was 12 years old. He was a refugee in Thailand until he came to the United States at age 13.

When he was interviewed during the first study, he was 16 years old, had been in the United States three and one-half years, and was in the eleventh grade. He indicated that he sometimes had difficulty finishing his homework and sitting still in class. He had few symptoms at the original interview but did become angry and irritable with some specific questions about his current feelings. He stated that he had no problems thinking about Cambodia, but he had never before discussed anything that happened there. He did say that he had felt sad perhaps 50 percent of the time in the previous two years. He also became challenging and contradictory in some of his answers, both in Cambodian and English, and he appeared to be fighting to maintain control of possible tears. He showed some signs of anger in the interview and looked away and avoided contact while describing some early events in Cambodia. After originally appearing well mannered and smiling, he showed much more anger, criticism, and denial besides being visibly upset. At that time, however, he did not meet the criteria for PTSD but was diagnosed with intermittent depressive disorder.

He was interviewed again when he was 20 years old. By this time he had graduated from high school, was engaged to a Cambodian student, and had worked temporarily as a carpenter. He now lived with four other Cambodians and felt very comfortable in this arrangement. He had enough money to meet his needs, although he was currently unemployed. He continued to avoid any thoughts that would bring back memories of the Pol Pot time, saying only, "I hate him (Pol Pot)." There were no alcohol, drug, or legal problems.

He appeared much more mature in the second interview but continued to show a disinterest, a restriction of affect, and clear avoidance of certain memories. This young man, although clearly impaired in some ways by his symptoms, with an original diagnosis of intermittent depressive disorder, showed no such symptoms at follow-up. He was functioning well and seemed satisfied with his life, but he was using denial and avoidance to control some of his disturbing memories.

Case 2: L. lived a stable and happy life in Cambodia with four siblings and his parents prior to Pol Pot. During the Pol Pot regime his parents were placed in work camps and his father, who had been a jewelry dealer, died of starvation. He also lost an older sister (during childbirth) and a brother-in-law. L. had to work hard and lost about 30 pounds during this time. While in the same work camp for three years, he saw people starving and dying, but remembered no specific incidents.

In 1979 he escaped across the border into Thailand. He described the Thai soldiers as worse than the Pol Pot cadres. He was only in the Thai camp for two months with a brother-in-law and his mother before being brought to this country by "a church group."

At the first interview, he was 20 years old, in the eleventh grade, and had no problems in school adjustment. He had been living with a couple of friends, having moved away from the brother-in-law and mother. He appeared to be a friendly, outgoing, handsome young man with a ready smile and a full range of affect. He had few symptoms at that time—just some difficulty concentrating and a few occasional worries about learning English.

At follow-up three years later, he was living with his 60-year-old mother and other Cambodians in the same house. He was working and supporting himself and had no financial problems. His manner was friendly and he had a good command of English. However, he showed many more symptoms than previously. He repeatedly said that he tried to avoid thoughts and memories about Pol Pot because "they ruin my life." He was afraid that he might "kill people" if the thoughts took over. He also said, "They taught me to kill," and he continued to fear a resurgence of Pol Pot memories. He felt vulnerable to these memories when watching television or reading the newspaper, or even when alone. He said he was often irritable and suddenly angry, and had trouble on a daily basis concentrating on new work. He had a general feeling of inadequacy and a sense that he might "go crazy," which put him on guard and made him vigilant with people. He sometimes startled easily when people came up behind him. This occurred at least once a week.

At the follow-up interview, L. described a fantasy experienced two years before of being on a beach, seeing every battle he had seen in Cambodia, and imagining that he also saw his father. He also told of challenging his co-workers at times. He found it difficult to deal with people who were "looking for trouble." Sometimes he said he couldn't be sure he might not grab a knife or a stick in a violent impulse. The most difficult experience he described was a confrontation with a policeman "who talked to with me like I had no education."

This Cambodian man, who seemd to be doing well at the first interview with few symptoms, at follow-up showed added symptoms with more intrusive thoughts, avoidance behavior, and fear of losing control and doing violence. There was a hint also that he had violence done to him or perpetrated violence on others. Despite trying to make the American dream come true, he clearly was suffering more, had more symptoms, and was more impaired at the second interview.

Case 3: C. was a 16-year-old tenth grader when first seen. He spoke very good English, saying that he had learned some in the Thai refugee camp. During the first year of Pol Pot, he was allowed to stay with his family, Cambodian farmers. For two years he lived in a labor camp only a mile away. He escaped in the second year and was able to live with his family for another year.

During the Pol Pot years, he saw five or six people killed. He denied any personal grievance because he was careful to do whatever he was asked. He always had enough to eat and denied going long periods without food. During the time he was in camp, he had no family contact.

C. was able to leave Cambodia during the Vietnamese invasion and his entire family made their way to the border into Thailand. He stayed in a refugee camp for two years until a Cambodian uncle sponsored his move to the United States. He lived in Texas for a year and one-half before coming to Portland in 1983.

He described having nightmares and some reexperiencing of the labor camp under Pol Pot. He had trouble getting to sleep and worried about his future. For three years he was easily startled by noise, and intrusive thoughts about Cambodia kept him from concentrating on his studies. He described having less feeling for people he used to care about and losing interest in daily activities. He showed PTSD symptoms along with anxiety and depression. He was pessimistic and brooded about what had happened in the past, feeling inadequate and irritable. He had been bothered by these feelings of depression a good deal in the prior two years. It was easy to establish a relationship with C. because of his openness. He was given a clear diagnosis of PTSD.

At follow-up, C. was 19 years old and had just completed U.S. Army boot camp. When not in the army he lived with his family. He had unpleasant thoughts about Pol Pot but they occurred much less often than before. Occasionally, perhaps once a month, unpleasant past thoughts intruded. There were no other symptoms of PTSD, anxiety, or depression. He enjoyed being in the army, being independent, and living away from parents and relatives. He appeared a serious-minded and impressive young man who had made an excellent adjustment in the past year. There was no evidence of impaired performance in any of his work or activities.

Case 4: V. was a 17-year-old high school sophomore when she was first seen. She had been living with a Cambodian foster mother. Before coming to the United States she had lived in a large city, where she attended school for four years. She was unsure what her father did but she knew he earned a good living. There were nine other children in the family.

When Pol Pot came to power, the father was captured and apparently committed suicide. V. was with him when he died. Her mother was in another camp and was never seen again, but it was later learned that she was executed. V. and three siblings were going to be executed but were spared, and V. was put with a group of older young people who were building dikes. She never saw any other family members for four years. She was never physically beaten. Pol Pot cadres, in addition to killing her mother, probably killed five brothers and sisters. Three younger siblings were killed as they were escaping and were hit with a mortar. She saw many people executed, "too many to count." An older sister was severely beaten and she refused to escape when the Vietnamese invaded. It was thought that she might still be in Vietnam, but no word was ever received from her.

V. did forced labor, building dikes, from morning to night. She lost so much weight during that time that she could not sit up. She said she looked like a skeleton. She tried to steal just enough food to live and work so that they would not kill her. Recalling her escape in 1979, she said that there were thousands who tried to get to the border, "corpses all over the place," starving, but she just kept going. She lived in a refugee camp for three years.

She came to the United States one year prior to her first interview. When seen at the first interview she had all of the PTSD symptoms including nightmares and difficulty falling asleep; she jumped and startled easily even at small noises. She had to be on guard and check the house security multiple times each day. She woke up frequently with nightmares and had been irritable for the past year. She had difficulty concentrating on her homework. She said she did not want to be around her friends but wanted to live alone and take care of only herself. She lost interest in most activities and did not want to do anything, feeling irritable and angry at times. She tried very hard to avoid anything that reminded her of Cambodia, saying it was unbelievable that she was still alive. She also had many symptoms of generalized anxiety and depressive and panic disorders.

In appearance, V. was an attractive young woman who seemed older than 17. She was serious and thoughtful throughout the interview, with little emotional expression but obviously engaged with the questions, and she found some relief talking about her experiences. Her concentration was good throughout. It was surprising, in view of her symptoms, that she was able to function moderately well and complete regular school activities.

Three years later she was seen at follow-up at her home in another state. She was a strikingly beautiful 21-year-old woman. She had spent two years going to secretarial school after leaving Portland, and had a fiance whom she had met in a Thai refugee camp. She said her major symptoms were better than they were before, but intrusive and startle symptoms were still present and occurred sometimes "too often." More than 50 percent of the time she had depressive symptoms, but there were days when she was "okay." She had panic attacks also. No diagnoses of other anxiety disorders were present. She had no problems with drugs or alcohol but "living in the United States was the most difficult thing I have experienced." Despite multiple symptoms she functioned well at work and had many friends and even taught classical Cambodian dance to students.

This young woman, with severe traumas and multiple symptoms, had been able to continue school, was working at the time of the second interview, but still had severe symptoms with a diagnosis of PTSD and depression with minimal overt behavioral impairment.

The studies described above provide dramatic evidence that trauma had profound and enduring effects on the subsequent development of these refugee children. Half of this group continued to receive an Axis 1 DSM-IIIR diagnosis despite the passage of time. Although the traumatic experience did not contribute to a delinquent or antisocial outcome, it did contribute to a fluctuating profile of PTSD or depression.

WAR AND DISRUPTIONS OF ATTACHMENTS IN EARLY LIFE

The Pol Pot regime in Cambodia deliberately fractured families by separating parents from children, putting them in different work camps. Some of the developmental consequences of these early disruptions are now beginning to be observed in clinical and social settings.

Both in our recent clinical work and in conversations with teachers in English as a Second Language programs, we have seen some Cambodian adolescents who are showing oppositional or conduct traits. These students are less respectful in class, take their studies less seriously, and have been experimenting with alcohol and drugs. We do not as yet have epidemiological data on this group of students, but hope to explore this population in the near future.

Our hypothesis about why such outcomes are now appearing is a developmental one. We postulate that this later group had developmental attachments fractured by the war at an early stage. Unlike the previous students who had roughly eight years of normal Cambodian family life prior to Pol Pot, these Cambodian adolescents had a much shorter period of early stability prior to the disruptions of Pol Pot. Some were born in the camps and raised by surrogate parents. Others were separated from parents prior to the age of two years.

The disruption of early, vital attachment relationships between children and their caretakers comprises one of the hidden tragedies of war. Parents (caretakers) became so distraught, distressed, or otherwise symptomatic by war that they were only marginally capable of responding to the day-to-day needs of young children. This further attenuated the attachment relationship. With the lack of attachment and cultural stability, guidance, and restraints, the stage had been set for later antisocial behavior. The following two cases seen since 1986 are given in illustration.

Case 5: P., a 14-year-old Cambodian girl, was brought by her mother to the clinic because of defiant behavior at home. She had been running away from home for two or three days at a time, not divulging to her mother where she had been. At school she was described as provocative and easily angered. She had been expelled on two occasions for fighting. Over the next year, she was charged twice with shoplifting. She also seemed to have considerable amounts of money, the source of which could never be determined. Whenever upset, she would tell her mother, "You are not my mother. I don't belong here."

At interview sessions, P. usually dressed all in black, claiming, "This is the Asian way." She was often dressed precociously, with excess jewelry and makeup. She had fluctuating ideas about her identity. She accused her mother of trying to raise her as a Cambodian when she was an "American." Yet at other times she drew her attention to her distinct Cambodian identity.

P.'s mother indicated that she had been separated from P. at the time of the Pol Pot takeover (when P. was one year old). P. was raised in one work camp with her grandmother while her mother lived and worked in another. At the end of the war the grandmother died suddenly of food poisoning and P.'s care was returned to her mother.

P.'s earliest memory was the death of her grandmother when she was four years old. She had no conscious memories of the Pol Pot camp. Her father was a soldier and his whereabouts were unknown. He was most likely executed at the beginning of the Pol Pot regime. A younger sibling, age six years, was doing well.

Attempts at both individual and family therapy were not successful in easing the tension between mother and daughter. P. repeated her assertion throughout that she did not "belong" at home. She finally ran away from home and was placed in an American foster home where she became more settled. She expressed no wish to return home.

Case 6: K. was evaluated at age 17 years in prison while awaiting trial on charges of murdering three Cambodian children, two of them quite young. K. gave little information about his previous life in Cambodia, although he appeared tense when we discussed it. He had few memories of his father and mother and perhaps two older brothers. He remembered leaving the city and going into the farm camp when he was about four years old. He did have a few strong images of his mother, whom he described as "very skinny" much of the time. She probably died of starvation. There is no further information on what happened to the rest of his family.

He was given to a woman called an aunt and stayed on and off with her during the Pol Pot regime from 1975 to 1979. Apparently for the last two years (1978 and 1979), he was in a camp of children six years of age and older.

He worked long and hard at that time and had little sleep. He saw many bodies and was aware of people dying, "sometimes two or three a day," probably from starvation. He denied any direct threats, although he was severely disciplined once for missing work.

After the Vietnamese invaded, he was reunited with his "aunt" and went to Thailand. It was a difficult time during which he was beaten by the aunt's husband. He then moved on to another family who had also just come out of Cambodia. They later had two children. K. was unofficially adopted by this family, and they came to the United States in 1981.

He said that many problems started at that time, with a lot of altercations and threatened beatings by his new parents. There seemed to be rigid rules and ongoing conflicts. He described having more violent fantasies for several years about hurting them. During that time, he described having many depressed feelings that would come and go. He said he felt suicidal much of the time and made one suicide attempt. His situation was alleviated somewhat when he moved out of that household into an American family's home. However, he felt increasingly isolated and taken advantage of there. These reactivated some previous memories of his adopted family. He made few friends in school, always felt like a loner, and had no one he could talk to, but he manifested no overt behavior problems.

One day he left class and went to his adopted family's home, brutally killing the three children. He was later convicted of this crime. While awaiting sentencing in prison, he concealed a fatal dose of medication from his guards and committed suicide.

CONCLUSION

The tragedy of Cambodia did not end with the cessation of the Pol Pot regime in 1979. The victims continue to suffer the effects of massive trauma, loss of country, and refugee status. Old and young both were affected. For the older patients the effects have left many psychiatrically impaired and have required a long-term treatment approach. We are just beginning to understand the effects of the Cambodian tragedy on the younger Cambodians, few of whom have become psychiatric patients. From our studies of high school students, we now know that PTSD symptoms affected about half of the students five years after the worst trauma ended. Depressive symptoms were even more common. Follow-up of these students three years later indicated that PTSD symptoms were still present in about half but the prevalence of depressed symptoms had diminished. Some students improved during this time but others developed symptoms for the first time. The avoidance symptoms, most commonly taking the form of refusing to think about the past, remained present in virtually all of the students. The case histories illustrate the variety of forms the symptoms and coping styles take in these young people as they grow into adulthood. The effects of such massive trauma on children is long-term and for many will show a variable course with intrusive symptoms periodically appearing in the individual's life. We recently have become aware of more antisocial behaviors being displayed by Cambodian students who were traumatized at an early age, beginning before the age of 12. It is possible that early trauma with the disruption of normal attachments leaves one vulnerable to later antisocial behavior. As we study Cambodians who were traumatized at an early age, we may gain more information about this phenomenon—yet another effect of massive trauma.

REFERENCES

Ablin, D. A., and Hood, M. (eds.) (1987). *The Cambodian Agony*. Armonk, N.Y.: M. E. Sharpe.

American Psychiatric Association. (1987). *Diagnostic and Statistical Manual of Mental Disorders*, 3rd ed. rev. Washington, D.C.: Author.

Beck, A. J., Ward, G. H., Mendelson, M., Mork, J. E., and Erbangh, J. K. (1961). An inventory for measuring depression. *Archives of General Psychiatry, 4*, 561–571.

Becker, E. (1986). *When the War Was Over*. New York: Simon and Schuster.

Boehnlein, J. K., Kinzie, J. D., Rath, B., and Fleck, J. (1985). One year follow-up study of posttraumatic stress disorder among survivors of Cambodian concentration camps. *American Journal of Psychiatry, 142*, 956–960.

Hawk, D. (1982). The killing of Cambodia. *New Republic, 198,* 17–21.

Kinzie, J. D. (1986). Severe posttraumatic stress disorder among Cambodian refugees: Symptoms, clinical course and treatment. In J. H. Shore (ed.), *Disaster Stress Studies: New Methods and Findings.* Washington, D.C.: American Psychiatric Press.

Kinzie, J. D., Fredrickson, R. H., Ben, R., Fleck, J., and Karls, W. (1984). Posttraumatic stress disorder among survivors of Cambodian concentration camps. *American Journal of Psychiatry, 141,* 645–650.

Kinzie, J. D., Sack, W., Angell, R., Clarke, G., and Ben, R. (1989). A three year follow-up of Cambodian young people traumataized as children. *Journal of American Academy of Child and Adolescent Psychiatry, 28*(4), 501–504.

Kinzie, J. D., Sack, W., Angell, R., Manson, S., and Rath, B. (1986). The psychiatric effects of massive trauma on Cambodian children: I. The children. *Journal of American Academy of Child Psychiatry, 25,* 370–376.

Robins, L. N., Helzer, J. E., Croughan, J., and Ratcliff, K. S. (1982). NIMH. Diagnostic interview schedule (DIS) Wave 2. St. Louis, Mo.: Washington University School of Medicine.

Sack, W., Angell, R., Kinzie, J. D., and Ben, R. (1986). The psychiatric effects of massive trauma on Cambodian children: II. The family, the home, and the school. *Journal of American Academy of Child Psychiatry, 25,* 377–383.

Shaffer, D., Gould, M. S., Brasic, J., Ambronsini, P., Fisher, P., Bird, H., and Aluwahlia, S. (1983). A children's global assessment scale (CGAS). *Archives of General Psychiatry, 40,* 1228–1231.

Spitzer, R. L., and Endicott, J. (1979). *Schedule for Affective Disorders and Schizophrenia: Lifetime Version,* 3rd ed. New York: New York Biometrics Research Division, New York Psychiatric Institute.

Weissman, M. N., Scholomabas, D., and John, K. (1981). Assessment of social adjustment. *Archives of General Psychiatry, 38,* 1250–1258.

Zilberg, N. J., Weiss, D. S., and Horowitz, M. J. (1982). Impact of Event Scale: A cross validation study and some empirical evidence supporting a conceptual model of stress response syndromes. *Journal of Consulting Clinical Psychology, 50,* 407–414.

6   Trauma and Adaptation: The Case of Central American Children

CONCHITA M. ESPINO, Ph.D.

Migration is a stressful process, challenging the resources of those who choose to undergo it. When it is accompanied by economic hardship, illegal status, and a physically dangerous environment, as is the case for many Central American families, the level of stress often exceeds the individual's capacities. For the children in these families, the added trauma of exposure to violence and prolonged separation from parents, who often arrive in the United States years prior to them, is exceedingly debilitating. Many normal developmental conflicts become unmanageable. Parents who themselves are experiencing high levels of anxiety and depression are unable to provide the support and structure needed to master the challenge.

Case 1: An 11-year-old boy from El Salvador named Douglas described fighting between soldiers and guerrillas around his home, which frequently required that the family abandon the home and hide. He reported that bombs would fall in his backyard and initially denied that anyone was hurt. After a long pause he said that "when they would come out of hiding there were only dead people." He proceeded to say, "One day there were three men by the house, one dead, one alive and one begging for water with all his insides hanging out. There were many asking for water. This would happen when there was fighting or when someone was killed by an enemy. They would come and dump them on the street and there they stayed until they died or their mothers came to get them." He then told how his grandfather was killed "just as he had caught a fish." It is unclear what this meant to Douglas but it suggests the intrusion of violence into an otherwise pleasant, routine activity.

Douglas admitted to remembering traumatic events when he did not want to, for example, the sound of a motorcycle brought back a vivid memory of a man who had been shot and whom he had seen crash to the ground. When he did his school work, "some things came out right and others came out wrong" because of thoughts he had about his grandmother being left back home. Douglas was aware that he had recounted all this in a monotone that "sounded like Frankenstein."

Douglas showed extremely constricted affect and seemed anxious. Throughout the interview he tapped the desk with his pencil in a slow, compulsive manner. The interview also showed that Douglas was at least of average intelligence, and had good reality testing and considerable self-awareness. He also had gradually developed trust in the interviewer after having shown guardedness initially.

Douglas had not been referred for treatment nor was he identified by teachers or parents as needing any sort of intervention. His poor school performance was attributed to his lack of knowledge of English and lack of formal education.

HISTORICAL BACKGROUND AND DESCRIPTION OF THE POPULATION

Estimates of the size and composition of the population of Central American families who have immigrated to the United States since the mid-1970s have been made by several demographers but are based on very limited data due to the largely undocumented status of the immigrants. In the Washington metropolitan area, three recent analyses of the population are available: the Comprehensive Technologies International (CTI) study (Beltrán, 1981), and the analyses of Grier and Grier (1983) and Martindale, Espino, and Berry-Caban (1986). From these studies certain characteristics can be surmised. For example, the Central American immigrant, although younger than the average American, may be slightly older than other Hispanics. There are also a larger number of females among this population in comparison with other immigrant groups. In fact, single women or women separated from their children are likely to be the vast majority of the new entrants. These new immigrant families also report a smaller percentage of children and a smaller percentage of households headed by women than their counterparts in the United States of Spanish origin. The median number of years of education of the adult women in one study (Martindale, Espino, and Berry-Caban, 1986) was 9. Forty percent of the sample in that same study had completed sixth grade levels of education or less.

This population of undocumented immigrants lived off their income and did not receive any federal income supplement, though the Women, Infant, and Children (WIC) program for infants and pregnant women was available to them. Employment was found in low-wage service jobs, mainly housekeeping and janitorial services. High rates of school enrollment (at one point in Washington, D.C., 20 new students per week began school) pressured the school boards of many counties in the Washington metropolitan area to develop bilingual programs to screen new students and place the large influx of immigrant children in special English as a Second Language (ESL) classrooms. Although these children show significant academic delays, the school board policy maintains that regardless of children's educational delay, they cannot be placed excessively below their expected grade level, which would create strains on both pupils and teachers.

Sociocultural Environment

Although there are a variety of subgroups within the Central American immigrant population that differ in their resources and capacities to adapt to life in the United States, certain generalizations can be made based on clinical observations and data collected for clinical purposes. Unpublished community surveys suggest that a majority of the population is from rural areas and has received little formal education. In the United States they have been forced to work long hours and live in overcrowded homes in the inner cities. This combination of factors often results in several conditions affecting the development of the children they bring with them.

According to a community survey done in Washington (Espino, Berry-Caban, and Gimenez, 1986) there is a very high incidence of neglect in this population. Their impoverished living conditions have resulted in poor supervision of children, physically dangerous environments, inadequate health care, and older siblings being burdened with adult responsibilities that interfere with their schooling and emotional development. Overcrowding has led to disruptions in sleep and exposure to sex and violence that is both overstimulating and threatening. Furthermore, their families are often highly unstable interpersonally and conflict-ridden due to the blending of families as a result of immigration patterns and the formation of new families when children from prior marriages are sent for, creating step- and half-sibling combinations. The rivalries between siblings, as well as between parents, are often highly emotionally charged. This home environment is not conducive to healthy emotional or cognitive development.

Education

According to a study of Central American children's academic and cognitive functioning (Espino et al., 1987) significant delays were observed. Among the sample of children ($n = 87$) who participated in this study,

Table 6.1. Group Means for Age, Years in the United States and Years of Formal Education Missed in the United States

Variable Name	Mean	Standard Deviation	Range	(Minimum–Maximum)
Age	11.8	2.25	9	(7–16)
Years in United States	3.19	2.39	9	(0–9)
Years of Formal Education				
Missed in the United States	−4.05	3.01	10	(0– −10)

35 percent were placed two or more years below their expected grade level by the board of education, in spite of the policy dictating that children be placed no more than 1 year behind. Table 6.1 indicates that when these children were given a school achievement test (in Spanish), 72 percent scored a two-or-more-year delay in reading and 73 percent scored this same delay in mathematics. It can also be seen that there is a large percentage of children who are behind fifth, sixth, or seventh grade levels in reading and math. These are adolescents who are reading at first- and second-grade levels. We may speculate that the level of stress and difficulties in adaptation for these youngsters is dangerously high and we may suspect that they are at risk for substance abuse and delinquency.

Once a child or adolescent reaches this level of academic delay, the motivation for school achievement is very poor and the loss of self-esteem and shame associated with any effort to perform or gain school-related skills is often great. Alternative behaviors involving pre-delinquent activities that mask these deficits become more attractive. Nevertheless, the youngster is impaired in his or her ability to read and interpret cues, in the ability to gain necessary information for making judgments, and in the capacity to master many activities of urban life. Youths are excluded by these deficits from participating in many activities that their peers who do have age-appropriate reading and mathematics skills engage in. Mastery of verbal skills that allow a youngster to interact with adults from a wide range of socioeconomic groups are also unavailable to them, thus limiting the area of the city and the type of activities in which they feel comfortable. Therefore a tendency to stay in a group and to function within a limited, familiar territory is enhanced.

Statement of the Problem

We suspected that traumatic experiences inhibited cognitive functions and curtailed adaptive resources of the children, leading to academic delays above and beyond those that could be accounted for by a lack of proficiency in English. Knowing that exposure to war violence and traumatic separation from parents occur frequently among Central American immigrant children, we decided to study various aspects of these traumas and their consequences. Several issues are involved regarding the impact of these traumas on the child's adaptive resources, for example, how it affected intellectual functioning (and cognitive functioning), whether symptoms of PTSD could be observed in children exposed to war violence, and if the impact of prolonged separation from parents could be measured.

In our work with a large group of Central American children in Washington, D.C., we designed a study that attempted to address some of these concerns and document the impact of the trauma these youngsters had experienced. In spite of the limitations of standardized psychological tests when used with minority populations, we chose to evaluate the level of intellectual functioning of Central American children using several instruments measuring their IQ, their academic achievement, and various other cognitive functions.

In addition, we developed rating scales to measure exposure to violence and post-traumatic stress disorder (PTSD) symptoms, as well as a method for scoring formal education in the United States and in the country of origin.

The purpose of the study was, first, to identify each child's degree of exposure to violence; second, to determine the presence or absence of PTSD symptomatology; and finally, to evaluate the relationship of both to the child's performance on tests of cognitive functioning. Separation from parents was treated in a similar manner: identifying the degree of separation, then the presence of PTSD symptoms, and finally its impact on cognitive functioning.

Some controversy exists concerning what constitutes a "trauma" as well as how children "respond to trauma." The original definition given by Freud (1923/1959) is based on the concept that a *trauma* is any excitation powerful enough to break through the stimulus barrier of the ego. Kris (1956) proposed that the concept of *strain trauma* be included so that the effects of long-term exposure to deprivation or noxious situations would be recognized as traumatic. Alternatively, Khan (1963) proposed the term *cumulative trauma* to connote the effect of the mother's failure to function as a protective shield. These definitions are consistent with Greenacre's (1967) definition of trauma as any condition that seems unfavorable, noxious, or drastically injurious to the development of the child. On the other hand, Anna Freud (1946), Rangell (1976), and Krystal (1978) reject these broader definitions of trauma and suggest that an essential characteristic of a trauma is that it be an experience that overwhelms the ego and produces painful effects (Green, 1983).

Green (1983) made a distinction between shocking traumatic events, which damage the receptive, processing, and integrative aspects of the ego, and cumulative trauma, which impairs affective development and ego functions involving self-preservation, establishment of object relationships, and identifications. He stated that "cumulative trauma would also adversely affect the long-term shaping of ego defenses, determining character formation, and would interfere with mastery and cognitive development" (p. 151).

Several studies have reported the effects of specific traumas on children, such as children exposed to catastrophic situations (Frederick, 1985), kidnapping (Terr, 1983), and physical abuse (Green, 1983). Research has also been conducted on children exposed to the violence of war in France (Mercier and Despert, 1942), Spain (Coromina, 1943), Israel (Ziv and Israel, 1973), and Central America (Arroyo, 1985). In a summary of his findings and a review of the literature on children traumatized by physical abuse, Green (1983) reported that in a sample of 60 abused children, 25 percent were found to be moderately or severely mentally retarded. He cites Martin et al. (1974) and Morse et al. (1970), who also report similar intellectual impairment in abused children. Specific cognitive impairments in the area of speech and language disorder have also been reported (Elmer and Gregg, 1967; Kempe, 1976; Martin, 1972). Nevertheless, Green (1983) notes that children who have experienced neglect and deprivation without being physically abused demonstrate the same degree of cognitive impairment as the abused sample.

Terr's (1983) study of the Chowchilla, California school bus kidnapping suggests that children's response to trauma may differ significantly from that of adults and that the symptoms of PTSD are not always manifested in children. Terr found the following: (1) children ages three or four years do not become amnesiac; (2) children, as opposed to adults, do not demonstrate psychic numbing, except perhaps those who have been chronically abused; (3) children do not experience sudden, unexpected visual flashbacks that interrupt their behavior or disrupt their concentration, possibly due to conscious daydreaming which may partly block the intrusion of gruesome visions; (4) children's work performance rarely suffers for more than a few months after psychic trauma; (5) post-traumatic play and reenactment occur much more frequently in childhood; (6) time skew (distortions in sense of time when events occurred) is more common and more dramatically expressed in children; and (7) children hold a foreshortened view of the future. Terr (1983) also reports the tendency in children to report omens or ghosts in relation to trauma of loss.

In a study of Central American children, Arroyo (1985) found that in addition to the symptoms included in the PTSD syndrome, this population of children traumatized by war, poverty, separation, domestic violence, and abuse showed symptoms that varied according to their age groups. In the children whom they saw at the clinic, they found the young children were withdrawn, and had characteristic symptoms of regression with separation and anxiety in the presence of strangers, bedwetting, and loss of acquired skills. Latency-age children showed learning inhibitions and conduct problems as well as somatic complaints. Adolescents exhibited serious acting-out behavior including delinquency and out-of-wedlock pregnancies. Arroyo (1985) concluded that, "the multiple traumas seem to have caused a long-term impairment in remote memory. As their poor school performance implies, other cognitive functions were affected as well" (p. 114).

Green, Lindy, and Grace (1985), in conceptualizations of the clinical entity in PTSD, describes the phenomenology of "the alternating intrusion-numbing cycles of both pathological and non-pathological processing." They refer to Horowitz (1976), who proposed an information-processing model to account for the re-experiencing of phenomena in PTSD. They also delineate several factors influencing PTSD. Their model includes (1) the experience of the event (degree of bereavement, life threat, and the role of the survivor); (2) individual characteristics (i.e., coping style); and (3) the recovery environment. All three sets of factors affect post-traumatic cognitive processing and adaptation.

In our work we will attempt to operationalize some of the factors related to the experience of the event and to describe adaptation within the narrow range of cognitive functioning.

In this study the effect of exposure to war violence was isolated from the other traumas to see if it results in specific symptoms of PTSD. The type and extent of trauma and the presence or absence of various PTSD symptoms was correlated. Further, several questions were asked, such as: Is there a specific effect of exposure to war violence that manifests itself in cognitive deficits as measured by standardized tests? Is the effect of separation from parents similar to the more acute trauma of exposure to violence?

METHOD

A combined approach of relying on standardized psychological tests and clinical interviewing techniques was employed. In addition, an attempt was made to quantify the data from the clinical interviews through the development of various checklists and indices. All interviews were conducted in the same setting by one interviewer and were taped so that various raters could score them. Two raters scored all the scales for each subject and a third investigator administered and scored all standardized tests.

SUBJECTS

The subjects were 87 Hispanic children who participated in various activity groups at a community agency in Washington, D.C. Some of the children were referred by the schools because they were experiencing behavioral or academic difficulties. Others responded to outreach efforts for group therapy, and a large number were recruited to participate in a summer art project which culminated in an exhibition at the Organization of American States (OAS). For that project children were encouraged to bring siblings and neighbors. This gave us a base of 100 children, of whom 87 participated in the study. The average age was 11.8 years and the children had been in the United States an average of three years.

INSTRUMENTS

Standardized administration of the Weschler Intelligence Scale for Children, Revised (WISC-R), Bender Gestalt, and Wide Range Achievement Test were followed. Scoring was also standardized and the Koppitz (1963) scoring method for the Bender Gestalt was used.

Adapted standardized administration for the Comprehensive Test of Basic Skills (CTBS) was employed. Both the reading and the mathematics parts were administered, separated by a 20-minute rest period. The groups were much smaller and more informal than the usual classroom setting in which the tests were given. Because of the limited formal education background of the children they were often administered a test one level lower than that expected for their age, which was very often more consistent with their present grade placement. Every decision was based on the principle of allowing the child to obtain the most favorable score possible.

INDICES AND CHECKLISTS DEVELOPED FOR THIS STUDY

Indices of Formal Education

Due to the varied and often limited background of formal education of the children and its importance as a confounding variable in measuring the relationship between trauma and cognitive functioning, we were very careful to measure as accurately as possible each child's experience with formal education in his or her own country and in the United States. Because parents who were living in the United States at the time their children were still living in the country of origin could not tell us exactly what grades their children attended or with what frequency they attended school, we devised a formula to estimate formal education in the country of origin. Two different indices to reach an accurate measure of formal education were necessary, one for formal education in country of origin and the other for formal education in the United States.

Index of Formal Education in the United States. This is a measure of how many years of formal education in the United States a child has missed in comparison to a child born and raised in the United States of the same age. It is presumed that a child arriving in the United States at age 13 years and having gone to school one year here has missed more U.S. formal education than a child arriving at age eight and having gone to school one year here, since the former should have attended school for a longer period of time than the latter. The index is computed by calculating the grade in which the child should be given his or her age, subtracting the number of years he or she has gone to school in the United States, and then placing a minus sign in front. In the above-mentioned example, then, the 13-year-old would receive a score of -7 and the 8-year-old would receive a score of -2.

Index of Formal Education in Country of Origin. This measure is an estimate of the quantity of formal education in the country of origin. Many children attended irregularly or had long-term disruptions in their schooling while others attended school very regularly. Since parents were unable to provide accurate information, we used a table of random numbers, picked two grades (specifically first and third), and (keeping those grades in mind), we asked parents to state if the child (1) often missed school for long periods of time, (2) went infrequently but without missing long periods of time, or (3) attended frequently. If the child had attended both first and third grade the average score was determined, always rounded up.

Exposure to Violence Index

To operationalize the trauma associated with war violence we developed a 12-item index based on the first five interviews (Figure 6.1). The items included general experiences such as witnessing maneuvers and bombing and specific experiences such as witnessing a family member being killed, as well as actual assault or trauma to the child. This index would

Figure 6.1. Clinical rating scale for exposure to war violence (based on structured interview with child)

Subject No. _____

	YES	NO
1. *Heard* bombs or shooting or the movement of troops in their town or nearby. Saw soldiers practicing maneuvers or target practicing.	—	—
2. *Heard* of soldiers or guerrillas engaging in specific actions such as raiding a house, taking food or clothing, or interrogating someone. This may include pressure to join the armed forces.	—	—
3. *Heard* of soldiers or guerrillas engaging in specific actions such as killing or raping or actual kidnapping.	—	—
4. *Saw* a person who was not a family member injured or traumatized by the war.[a]	—	—
5. *Saw* a person who was not a family member killed or dead as a result of the war.	—	—
6. *Heard* of a family member injured or traumatized as a result of the war.	—	—
7. *Heard* of a family member being killed as a result of the war.	—	—
8. *Saw* a family member injured or traumatized as a result of the war.	—	—
9. *Saw* a family member killed or dead as a result of the war.	—	—
10. *Child* was threatened by or temporarily held hostage by guerrillas or soldiers or was present when family was forced to cooperate against their will with guerrillas or soldiers by giving food or shelter.	—	—
11. *Child* was injured or traumatized by guerrillas or soldiers.	—	—
12. *Child* had a traumatic border crossing which was experienced by the child as dangerous or frightening.	—	—
Global assessment of degree of exposure to war violence.	1 2 3 4 5	

[a]This category includes the general disorganization that might take place in a town as a result of fighting. This may include barroom brawls and violence among town members.

then be scored by the interviewer and by a second person who heard the tape. Both raters also scored each child's experience on a five-point global measure that was used to sort the children into five groups, from no exposure to violence to severe and specific exposure to violence. Inter-rater correlations were calculated to determine how reliably a child's experience of war trauma could be assessed from the interview.

Indices of Separation

Several measures of separation were computed. These measures involved the number of years during which a child had been separated from (1) his or her mother, (2) his or her father, and (3) from both at the same time. In addition, the child's age at the time of these separations was also determined.

PTSD Symptom Checklist

This is a 15-item checklist which includes the symptoms in *Diagnostic and Statistical Manual*, 3rd ed. revised (*DSM III-R*) as well as some of the findings recently reported in research with children (Figure 6.2). The checklist was completed by the interviewer based on the information gathered from the parent interview, the child's own report, and the interviewer's own observations of the child.

PROCEDURE

Information was gathered from four different sources. First, a parent interview based on a structured questionnaire yielded most of the demographic data, pertinent social and individual history (i.e., years of separation and schooling), and information regarding traumatic experiences that each child had experienced as far as the parent knew. The parents were also asked about symptoms observed in the child, particularly nightmares, regression, exaggerated startle response, etc.

Second, a structured, taped interview with the child was conducted. The interview was designed to elicit experiences related to war violence or other traumatic experiences and to explore the presence of PTSD symptoms.

Each interview with a parent and each taped interview with a child was done by one single investigator. Thus one individual elicited both the exposure to violence information and the PTSD symptomatology. This was necessary due to the need to build trust and develop rapport with the children and parents. Finally, two raters listened to the taped interviews and each separately scored the exposure to violence and the PTSD symptom checklist. Although each rater scored all the children on both scales, this was not done sequentially, so that when rating the last part of the interview, which addressed the PTSD symptoms, the rater was unlikely to remember the subject's score on the exposure to violence scale since she had scored about 80 subjects in between. In order to provide inter-rater reliability on both scales four separate raters

Figure 6.2. Clinical rating scale for symptoms related to post-traumatic stress disorder

Subject No. _____

(Based on Child's Report)	YES	NO
1. Have you remembered without wanting to violent things that happened?	—	—
2. Have you had dreams about violent things that happened?	—	—
3. Have you had nightmares?	—	—
4. Have you suddenly felt that the same thing is happening again?		

(Based on observation and parent interview)		
5. Child seemed to lose interest in activities that she or he used to like.	—	—
6. Child feels detached from others.	—	—
7. Child shows little affect.	—	—
8. Child reports recurrent memories of trauma(s).	—	—
9. Child appears to be hyperalert and to have an exaggerated startle response.	—	—
10. Child has sleep disturbances.	—	—
11. Child demonstrates guilt about survival.	—	—
12. Child has memory impairment or concentration difficulties.	—	—
13. Child avoids activities that remind him or her of trauma. (The child may state that he or she wishes to avoid places or events that are associated with the trauma.)	—	—
14. Child's symptoms increase by remembering trauma.	—	—
15. There is a history of loss of function (i.e., speech, toilet training, or separation-individuation milestones).	—	—
Level of anxiety during interview	1 2 3 4 5	
Level of depression during interview	1 2 3 4 5	

would have been needed. Because of lack of funds, this was not possible, so that a certain amount of bias had to be tolerated in this case.

On the other hand, all other measures were administered and scored by a third investigator who had no access to the taped interviews or the scored checklists. Individual tests were administered in Spanish, including the WISC-R, the Bender Gestalt Test, and the Draw-a-Person Test. The Wide Range Achievement Test (reading and spelling parts only) was administered individually in English.

Table 6.2. Mean Score for Each Group on Post-traumatic Stress
        Disorder (PTSD) Symptom Checklist[a]

Variable: Global Score of Exposure to Violence	Mean No. of Symptoms on Checklist
Group	
1	0.6250
2	1.6007
3	2.0000
4	1.5000
5	4.4167

[a]For explanation of groups, see text.
$F = 7.9197$.
$P = <.0001$.

RESULTS

Exposure to Violence and PTSD Symptoms

A group of children who had been exposed to war violence more than others was identified by employing the exposure to war violence scale. The sample was sorted on the basis of a global score of 1 to 5 given by the raters, with group 1 being composed of children not exposed to war violence, while children in group 5 had been exposed to the most intense violence. Of the sample, 29.7 percent were assigned to group 1, 14.9 percent to group 2, 18.9 percent to group 3, 12.6 percent to group 4, and 21.6 percent to group 5. The mean number of PTSD symptoms for each group was computed showing statistically significant difference among the groups (Table 6.2). Thus the instrument that was developed to identify symptoms of PTSD proved useful and showed a strong correlation with exposure to war violence scores. Children who had been exposed to mutilation or death or had been kidnapped themselves (group 5) showed a statistically higher number of PTSD symptoms than the other children in the sample. Group 1, who had not been exposed to war violence, showed almost no symptoms. All groups differed significantly from group 5.

Inter-rater reliability for the exposure to violence scale was very high for the scale as a whole ($r = .96$) and the reliability using the Kuder-Richardson measure of internal consistency was $r = .6785$. Certain items, for example, item 6 (Figure 6.1), "Heard of a family member injured or traumatized as a result of the war" had an inter-rater reliability of $r = .6764$. Item 7, "Heard of a family member being killed as a result of the war," had an $r = .4960$ and item 10, "Child was threatened by or temporarily held hostage by guerrillas or soldiers," had an r value of .65. It is interesting to note that at face value these are also the items that might be considered to signal the most traumatizing experiences excluding, of course, item 11, "Child was injured or traumatized by guerrillas or soldiers," which was not reported by any of the children.

Internal consistency of the PTSD–related symptom checklist (Figure 6.2) was computed using alpha coefficients and attained an alpha of 0.8537. Five items yielded low correlations with the rest of the other items and it is important to note what these items were. These were items 2, 4, 9, 12, and 14.

— Dreams about violent things

— Suddenly feeling that the same thing is happening again

— Child appears hyperalert

— Child has memory impairment or concentration difficulties

— Symptoms increase by remembering the trauma

It is unclear what the poor correlation of these items with the rest of the scale reflects. The low correlation of item 2 may simply reflect its lack of specificity. On the other hand, the other four items are important components of the definition of PTSD. It must be noted that *Diagnostic and Statistical Manual of Mental Disorders*, 3rd edition (*DSM-III*) requires that only one symptom evidencing the reexperiencing of the trauma, one symptom of numbing of responsiveness, and two symptoms of six listed in the third category be present for a positive diagnosis. Thus considerable variability in symptomatology is expected according to this definition.

Several items in the PTSD symptom checklist were reported with high frequency. For example, flashbacks were reported by about 13 percent of the group. This is in contrast to the findings reported by Terr (1983). Terr failed to find this symptom in the traumatized children she studied. On the other hand, symptoms associated with detachment or numbing of responsiveness or constricted affect were not identified frequently. This is consistent with Terr's findings of children traumatized in small groups. Exaggerated startle response was observed or reported by about 17 percent of the children. Sleep disturbances were reported by a large number of the children, and probably this symptom is not specific to PTSD.

Separation

Finally, prolonged separation from parents did not show a correlation with PTSD symptoms. We suspect that our measures, number of years separated from mother, from father, or from both, contained too much variability for such a small sample. Using age of first separation also proved not to be correlated to any of the PTSD symptoms. When we divided the sample into separated and not separated and made a dichotomous variable, we found significant differences. Looking at these data closely we noted that this division of the sample was exactly equivalent to group 1 versus groups 2, 3, 4, and 5 in the exposure to violence scale. That is, the same children who had not been exposed to war violence at all had also not been separated from their parents. Thus we felt it was most parsimonious to explain these results in light of the protective factor provided by the parents of these children rather than to any specific effect of separation.

Cognitive Development

Cognitive functioning as measured by the WISC-R, Bender Gestalt, figure drawing, and achievement tests proved to be related to trauma in a manner of greater complexity than this experimental design allowed for. The findings shown in Table 6.3 were reported.

1. Children not exposed to war violence *at all* scored about 10 points higher on the WISC-R full-scale IQ and the performance IQ tests than children who were exposed to war violence (see Table 6.3). Analysis of covariance showed that this significant difference was not due to years of formal education in the United States. At the same time, formal education in the United States is correlated with full-scale IQ and performance IQ. It is important to note the complexity of the relationship. That is, what appears to be a contradiction is actually the work of two factors working conjointly.

2. Children exposed to war violence scored about 10 points below the U.S. norm on the WISC-R, but this effect is most likely not *specific* to the trauma but is due to other intervening variables, since degree of war violence did not increasingly impact on cognitive functioning. This finding is in contrast to the relationship with PTSD symptoms in which the degree of war violence systematically affected the number of symptoms.

3. We were surprised to find that children exposed to war violence scored relatively closer to U.S. norms on the WISC-R than on achievement tests in Spanish or in English. That is, deficits were greater in achievement tests than in IQ tests. In addition, the difference between children exposed to war violence and children not exposed to war violence on achievement tests could not be accounted for by years of formal education. This pattern was similar to that found in the IQ tests. The greater deficit found in achievement tests versus IQ tests are measuring

Table 6.3. Group Means for WISC-R Full-Scale IQ

	Groups Based on Global Score on Exposure to Violence Scale				
	Group 1[a]	Group 2	Group 3	Group 4	Group 5
Full-scale IQ	101.4545	83.9091	86.5358	85.1111	84.0067

One-Way Analysis of Variance for WISC-R Full-Scale IQ
Analysis of Variance Table
Source of Variation Group

DF	Sum of Squares	Mean Squares	F-Value	Probability (Tail)
4	4,192.8837	1,038.2209	5.7852	.0005
65	11,777.4161	181.1910		

Exposure to Violence Group[a]	Probabilities for the T-Values				
	1	2	3	4	5
1	1.000				
2	0.008*	1.0000			
3	0.0023	0.6351	1.0000		
4	0.0031	0.8431	0.8076	1.0000	
5	0.0003*	0.9766	0.6296	0.8546	1.0000

Abbreviations: DF, degrees of freedom; F, frequency
[a]Group 1 = no exposure to war violence; group 5 = exposure to mutilation and death.
*$p = .001$.

something other than just school-based knowledge and skills. Thus, these children, although their IQ scores are depressed, have a much more marked deficit in school-based knowledge and skills. We can confidently state that severe deficits in academic skills were found, and have been discussed in this chapter.

These deficits were correlated to lack of formal education, but children protected from exposure to war were able to significantly compensate more effectively for the lack of formal education than children who were exposed to war violence. Sociocultural factors are likely responsible for this between-group difference within this population.

CONCLUSION

Correlation between exposure to violence and PTSD symptomatology was found. Symptoms reported by our population are consistent with previous findings except for flashbacks, which the children in this study reported. We feel confident that a diagnostic interview can reliably identify PTSD in children and that a rating scale of the type used in this study is useful for reporting purposes. We encourage the use of this diagnosis and expect further refinement in the identification of symptoms. Although some bias may have been introduced by the use of the same raters for both scales, the specificity that we found between exposure to violence and PTSD symptoms which did not exist between prolonged separation and PTSD symptoms adds to the impression that the relationship we found is valid as measured by the two checklists.

On the other hand, cognitive functioning as tapped by the psychological tests administered in the study seem to relate to trauma in a complex manner. The fact that children not exposed to war violence at all scored significantly higher than all other groups can be interpreted as a demonstration of the importance of a combination of factors that result in successfully protecting a child from trauma. The children in this group may actually belong to a slightly higher social class and may have had parents with slightly greater resources. The demographic data available were not sufficient to determine if this hypothesis can be sustained. Certain factors related to stability in the environment or the protective functions played by a caretaker seem to be conducive to intellectual development. We can only state our finding that the group of children scoring high on IQ and achievement tests were precisely those children who had been protected from exposure to war. Further, these children scored high in spite of lack of formal education in the United States. Further research is called for to identify what factors lead to such apparent strength of adaptive resources.

In summary, the 1980s have seen the immigration of Central American families primarily to three major U.S. metropolitan areas, Los Angeles, Washington, D.C., and Miami, Florida. Although accurate demographic or epidemiological data are not available, several areas of difficulties in adaptation can be noted. Families from war-torn areas arrive with the scars of traumas experienced in their country of origin as a result of exposure to violence and poverty. On their arrival they become part of the inner city working poor with the added anxiety of illegal status. The children, living in overcrowded, high-conflict homes, experience neglect and abuse. Marked educational delays further inhibit their capacity to adapt, resulting in loss of self-esteem and depression. A large percentage of these children are further cognitively and emotionally handicapped and can be diagnosed as having PTSD.

REFERENCES

American Psychiatric Association (1987). *Diagnostic and Statistical Manual of Mental Disorders*, 3rd ed. rev. Washington, D.C.: Author.

Arroyo, W. (1985). Children traumatized by Central American warfare. In S. Eth and S. Pynoos (eds.), *Post-traumatic Stress Disorders in Children.* Washington, D.C.: American Psychiatric Association.

Beltrán, C. M. (1981). Hispanic population and characteristics in the Washington, D.C., metropolitan area. Prepared for Radio WMDO, Radio Mundo by Comprehensive Technologies International.

Coromina, J. (1943). Repercussions of the war on children as observed during the Spanish Civil War. *The Nervous Child, 2,* 324–337.

Elmer, E., and Gregg, C. S. (1967). Developmental characteristics of abused children. *Pediatrics, 40,* 596–602.

Espino, C., Berry-Caban, C., and Giminez, S. (1986). Characteristics of hispanic families experiencing child abuse and neglect. Unpublished manuscript.

Espino, C., Sanguinetti, P., Moreno, F., Diehl, V., and Zea, M. D. (1987). Psychological testing of hispanic children: The role of war violence. Paper presented at the meeting of the American Psychological Association Meeting, New York, N.Y.

Frederick, C. (1985). Children traumatized by catastrophic situations. In S. Eth and S. Pynoos (eds.), *Post-traumatic Stress Disorders in Children,* pp. 71–99. Washington, D.C.: American Psychiatric Association.

Freud, A. (1946). *The Ego and the Mechanisms of Defense.* New York: International Universities Press.

Freud, S. (1959). Beyond the pleasure principle. In J. Strachey (ed. and trans.), *The Standard Edition of the Complete Psychological Works of Sigmund Freud,* vol. 18. London: Hogarth Press. (Original work published 1923.)

Green, A. H. (1983). Dimensions of psychological trauma in abused children. *Journal of American Association of Child Psychiatry, 22,* 231–237.

Green, B. L., Lindy, J. D., and Grace, M. C. (1985). Post-traumatic stress disorders: Toward DSM-IV. *Journal of Nervous and Mental Disease, 173*(7), 406–411.

Greenacre, P. (1967). The influence of infantile trauma on genetic patterns. In S. Furst (ed.), *Psychic Trauma,* pp. 108–153. New York: Basic Books.

Grier, E. S., and Grier, G. (1983). *Newcomers: Problems and Needs of Refugees and Other Recent Arrivals to the Washington Community: A Reconnaissance.* (Report prepared under a grant from the Community Foundation of Greater Washington.) Washington, D.C.: Greater Washington Research Center.

Helfer, R. E., McKinney, J., and Kempe, R. (1976). Arresting or freezing the developmental process. In R. E. Helfer and C. H. Kempe (eds.), *Child Abuse and Neglect: The Family and Community,* pp. 64–73. Cambridge, Mass.: Ballinger.

Horowitz, M. J. (1976). *Stress Response Syndrome.* New York: Jason Aronson.

Khan, M. (1963). The concept of cumulative trauma. *Psychoanalytical Study of the Child, 18,* 54–88.

Koppitz, E. M. (1963). *The Bender Gestalt Test for Young Children.* New York: Grune & Stratton.

Kris, E. (1956). The recovery of childhood memories. *Psychoanalytic Study of the Child, 11,* 54–58.

Krystal, H. (1978). Trauma and affect. *Psychoanalytic Study of the Child, 33,* 8–116.

Martin, H. P. (1972). The child and his development. In C. H. Kempe and R. E. Helfer (eds.), *Helping the Battered Child and His Family,* pp. 93–114. Philadelphia: J. B. Lippincott.

Martin, H. P., Breezly, P., and Conway, E. F. (1974). The development of abused children. *Advances in Pediatrics, 21,* 439–447.

Martindale, M., Espino, C., and Berry-Caban, C. (1986). Profile of the hispanic population in the Washington, D.C. metropolitan area. Unpublished manuscript.

Mercier, M. H., and Despert, J. L. (1942). Psychological effects of the war on French children. *Psychosomatic Medicine, 5,* 266–272.

Morse, W., Sahler, O. J., and Friedman, J. B. (1970). A three-year follow-up study of abused children. *American Journal of the Disturbed Child, 120,* 439–446.

Rangell, L. (1976). Discussion of the Buffalo Creek disaster: The course of psychic trauma. *American Journal of Psychiatry, 133,* 313–316.

Terr, L. (1983). Chowchilla revisited: The effects of psychic trauma four years after a schoolbus kidnapping. *American Journal of Psychiatry, 140,* 1543–1550.

Ziv, A., and Israel, R. (1973). Effects of bombardment on the manifest anxiety level of children living in Kibbutzim. *Journal of Consulting and Clinical Psychology, 40,* 287–291.

III SERVICE AND TREATMENT ISSUES

Refugee children represent both a special population, with unique treatment needs and service delivery requirements, and a subset of a much larger population of children with multiple needs, who require a comprehensive system of care. As discussed in the chapters of this section, if services are to be responsive to the special needs of refugee children, they must incorporate unique components, such as bilingually and biculturally trained staff, and culturally sensitive outreach to and linkages with the refugee community. At the same time, services for refugee children need to encompass the system design features necessary for effective service delivery for all children with multiple needs, namely, comprehensiveness, accessibility, flexibility, affordability, appropriateness, and coordination of services. This section focuses on the treatment and service needs that must be addressed if refugee children are to be helped in meeting the challenges posed by their past, present, and future.

In Chapter 7, Joseph Westermeyer describes situations that may lead to emotional problems in children and adolescents and then identifies common types of psychopathology among refugee children. Assessment strategies are outlined and a comprehensive treatment program described.

Margaret Leiper de Monchy summarizes in Chapter 8 the special problems refugee children have faced and identifies how these problems and needs must be integrated into the systems that are designed to serve refugee youth. Two model programs are described. De Monchy emphasizes the need for service providers to understand the problems of refugee children in order to do no harm and the importance of designing services that build on the strengths of these young people.

Timothy Ready reports in Chapter 9 on a follow-up study of a group of Central American youth who were enrolled in a school that provided an unusual degree of assistance and support. This study demonstrates the long-term impact that appropriate and comprehensive services can have for even the most troubled children.

In Chapter 10, Carolyn L. Williams discusses the need for prevention programs. She notes that few, if any, true primary prevention programs exist for refugee youth. She explores the reasons for this lack of effective prevention programming, and also discusses what primary prevention actually is. Examples are given and suggestions are made for models for primary prevention program development for this at-risk group.

.

7 Psychiatric Services for Refugee Children: An Overview

JOSEPH WESTERMEYER, M.D., M.P.H., Ph.D.

Refugee children generally adjust satisfactorily to their new resettlement communities. A popular stereotype is that, because they have survived the rigors of refugee flight, they are immune to social maladjustment and psychiatric disorders. Refugee children at increased risk for developing mental health problems include those without their families, children with brain damage from trauma or malnutrition, those in partial families, and those whose parents are psychiatrically or socially disabled. Assessment and care of these children involves special knowledge and skill. The purpose of this chapter is to describe these special issues in order to improve services for refugee children. Program planning for refugee children and their families, traumatized by war and violence, must take into account these special needs and approaches. The need for translators and outreach workers who are refugees themselves, the extra time required for cross-cultural assessment, and the high rate of brain damage in some groups must be considered in planning services and programs. These must be translated into such programmatic considerations as higher staff/patient ratio, hiring and training refugee staff, access to psychological testing and radiographic brain imaging, staff training, and increased cost per patient.

BACKGROUND

About 100 million people have fled their countries due to war, civil unrest, and political or religious persecution during the last 50 years. Aronson (1984) has estimated that 16 million people were either in transit or had recently been granted asylum in a foreign country during the early 1980s. About 1 percent of the American population is composed of refugees from World War II, the unsuccessful Hungarian and Czechoslovak revolutions, Cuba, Southeast Asia, the Middle East, East Africa, and Iran. In addition, as many as one million "illicit refugees" from Central America and elsewhere may currently live in the United States.

Some refugee flights have consisted largely of young single adults; the Hungarian and Czechoslovak flights are examples. Most large-scale flights involve children, however. At any one point in time, about half the refugees in the world are children and adolescents under the age of 18 years (Williamson, 1988). For example, among the first wave of 67,499 Vietnamese refugees in the United States, 46 percent were aged 0 to 17 years (Kelly, 1977).

Many categories of refugee children can be discerned. Some were refugees as children, but they are now adults. Others came to the United States as refugee children and are still minors at this time. Children born to refugee parents in the United States share many of the characteristics of refugee children, although they are not technically refugees. Depending upon the strictures of one's definitions, then, the number of "refugee children" in the United States may vary from a few hundred thousand to perhaps a few million individuals.

ASSESSMENT

Several aspects in assessing refugee children require special consideration. These fall into two general categories: (1) their past experience and background and (2) their current life within refugee families.

Children's Experience as Refugees

Child and adolescent development occurs along biological, psychological, social, and cultural lines. These developmental issues set the refugee child apart from the refugee adult: they are not merely smaller or younger versions of their refugee elders. Refugee experiences occur at a time when children are both more vulnerable in certain ways, as well as more adjustable and flexible. Refugee children therefore have some advantages over their elders in terms of acculturation to a new society. They also are heir to certain types of problems different from adults, such as loss of their parents at a time when they are dependent on them. Experiences such as malnourishment or brain trauma can have markedly different consequences for children as compared to adults. Refugee-related events that occur during adolescence or young adulthood can have effects that resemble those experienced by both younger children and adults (Carlin, 1979).

It is impressive that refugee children can experience and minimize *life-threatening situations* if their parents are in a position to support and protect them. The Polish-American sociologist Lopata (1975) reported that she gaily greeted her adolescent friends on her admission to a Nazi detention camp in Germany while her American-born mother struggled feverishly to exempt the family from the arriving cattle cars. Smyke (1988) described the response of an 8-year-old child fleeing Afghanistan with her physician parents. The child behaved as though the flight were an excursion or a camping trip. After several days of being hungry, cold, and tired, the daughter remarked, "I think we should go to a hotel now. I really need a bath and some clean clothes." A Hmong girl, later my foster daughter, spent several weeks trekking the mountains of northern Laos as her village sought escape from advancing North Vietnamese troops. They scrounged food from the forests as they went. On one occasion, they passed a Vietnamese army unit going in the opposite direction in the valley below—each side with weapons at hand. Aged 11 at the time, she perceived it as a great and glorious time: the family and neighbors forgot petty dissensions to work together; she slept in the midst of her family each night "with the beautiful stars above"; and the new sights and places were exciting to see. Leon et al. (1981), in a study of the postwar offspring of Holocaust survivors, found no evidence of gross psychopathology as assessed by the Minnesota Multiphasic Personality Inventory.

From birth children are ensocialized into their families' society. Certain lessons not learned in childhood may be extremely difficult or even impossible to learn later. For example, tonal language is learned readily in childhood but poorly in adulthood (Westermeyer and Westermeyer, 1977). Numerous attributes of personality, cognition, symbol, understanding, and value system are acquired readily in childhood but are acquired only with great difficulty later. These are learned at "the father's knee" or "the mother's breast" through observation and emulation of relatives in the intimacy of the family, through proverbs, scoldings, and rewards. This process is referred to as *ensocialization*. The refugee resettling as an adult thus misses this critical phase and always remains something of a stranger, a marginal person in the adopted homeland. Through American peers, teachers, and mass media, refugee children become ensocialized into American society in a way that their elders can never replicate.

Acculturation refers to the process of exchanging attributes of culture, although ordinarily the larger culture-in-situ donates these to the migrant while changing little in return. (Massive, concentrated refugee flights—such as the Cubans into south Florida—may serve as an exception.) This process refers to the acquisition of language, clothing, social and work skills, and other attributes that produce a "hyphenated American" (e.g., Irish-American, Japanese-American). Although not thoroughly an American culturally, the adult refugee or migrant can acquire knowledge, skills, and attitudes congenial to survival, a livelihood, citizenship, a rewarding lifestyle, and general social competence (accompanied by some social ineptitude or cultural dissonance).

Child and adolescent refugees differ from their adult peers in that they are simultaneously acculturating to the new society while being ensocialized within the family. For the infant under one year of age, the process may involve a bicultural ensocialization, to the culture at home and to the prevailing society. For the newly arrived older adolescent, the process mainly involves acculturation, with perhaps some ensocialization in high school, college, the Job Corps, or the military.

Causes of Psychiatric Disorder and Maladjustment

The factors listed here are not the only causes of maladjustment among refugee children. Genetic, constitutional, environmental, and biomedical conditions can and do contribute to such problems. These potential causes are especially apt to occur among refugee children, whereas they are infrequent among indigenous children.

Malnutrition and Infectious Disease. These conditions may occur in the chaos of refugee flight, when a balanced nutritious diet may not be available for days, weeks, or months. When refugee relief efforts first get underway, refugee camps may not provide adequate nutrition for several months. Lack of nutrition affects children more rapidly and more seriously than adults for three reasons. First, children and adolescents have a higher metabolic rate than adults, thus requiring more food per unit of body weight simply to remain alive. Second, food above and beyond basic metabolic needs is necessary for normal growth and development in children and adolescents. And third, children can suffer permanent biodevelopmental damage (e.g., brain damage, small stature) as a result of malnutrition.

Children are also more likely than adults to develop infectious disease under flight conditions, since they have not yet developed resistance as have adults. Exposed to crowded refugee conditions, poor sanitation, exposure to the elements, and exhaustion, the risk to infection is high (Hodson and Springthorpe, 1976). Many refugee children have lost siblings due to infectious disease, much as in the typical American family prior to 1920. Infections also contribute to malnutrition, since protein and other body stores used to fight the infection may not be replaced later (Olness, 1977). History of infection or malnutrition should lead to a consideration of brain damage as a cause for maladjustment, as in Case 1.

Case 1: A 12-year-old orphaned Hmong boy had been placed out of the home due to beatings by a grandmother, temper tantrums and disobedient behavior at home, and failing work in school. Teachers reported poor attention and concentration and constant motion in and about the classroom. His family had fled Laos when he was a newborn, and he had spent his first year of life in a refugee camp with poor nutrition and no medical services. On two occasions he had high spiking fevers accompanied by convulsions. Physical examination revealed obesity, poor coordination, dydiadochokinesia, and asymmetrical reflexes. Computerized testing showed poor attentionality and impulsivity. His IQ was 119. He responded well to an individualized school program, family counseling, and a 6-month course of methylphenidate.

Even after resettlement in the United States, malnutrition and infectious disease remain as threats for refugee children. Some refugee families do not provide adequate fruits and vegetables for their families, since these are more expensive than in Third World countries, whereas meat and grains are the same price or less in the United States. Subsequent development of diet-induced cardiovascular disease, as has occurred among Japanese-Americans (Marmot and Syme, 1976), poses a risk for later life. Immunizations may be avoided by parents unfamiliar with them. Refugee children may be at risk for contagious diseases carried by their elders and newly arriving relatives (e.g., hepatitis B, tuberculosis, shigellosis). Some pediatric conditions, such as chronically draining ear infections, may be viewed by parents as "normal" since nothing could be done for these problems in the country of origin. This parental attitude can lead to lifelong consequences, such as hearing impairment. Children may not be brought to medical attention in a timely fashion when refugee parents are suspicious or fearful of medical interventions, with subsequent risk to major complications.

Refugee children can have chronic conditions or carrier states infrequent among indigenous children. Examples include congenital hemoglobinopathies that result in chronic or acute anemias, and hepatitis B carrier status which carries the risk of subsequent hepatoma (Murray et al., 1988). Large family size, which has been correlated with shorter stature (Bogin and MacVean, 1981), is frequent in some refugee groups.

Physical Trauma. Refugee children may be victims of violence due to war injuries, beating, and even torture. This odious fact is often not appreciated by those assessing refugee children, with the result that injuries to the organ of adaptation and learning—the brain—are often missed, as in the following case.

Case 2: An eight-year-old Vietnamese boy was referred by his school because of misbehavior in the classroom and failure to acquire the English language. Evaluation by a pediatrician had been negative. The patient was otherwise bright, engaging, and socially skilled. On examination, the child had a well-healed 2-cm-long scar on his forehead and several frontal lobe release signs (i.e., palmomental, suck, snout, and rooting reflexes). On x-ray examination a 2-cm piece of shrapnel was observed in the frontal region. On directed history, the family reported that the child had been wounded during a mortar attack. Computed tomography (CT) scan and electroencephalogram (EEG) revealed extensive frontal lobe damage. Educational recommendations and family counseling were aimed at enhancing the adjustment of a child with frontal lobe syndrome.

Among several of our refugee children, traumatic brain damage occurred in the United States. Their parents—new to driving—had become involved in serious vehicular accidents. The children, who had usually not been placed in appropriate restraints, were seriously injured. Refugees should be instructed regarding the potential risks of vehicular accidents to their children and the need (often the legal imperative) for children to be restrained in vehicles.

Child Neglect and Abuse. This may not be expected among people whose cultures place high value on children, the parental role, and child raising skills. In the context of migration, resettlement, adjustment problems, and associated mental disorder, such problems unfortunately do occur. Some refugee children, especially unaccompanied minors, have been subject to physical or sexual abuse by foster families. Some have survived in Asia by engaging in prostitution (homosexual or heterosexual). As substance abuse has appeared and spread among refugee parents (i.e., alcoholism, opium addiction), refugee child abuse and neglect has increased appreciably.

Case 3: A fearful and maladaptive six-year-old Vietnamese boy was referred by the school. He described anal intercourse and other sexual activities with his "uncle" for "as long as I can remember." The "uncle" had obtained the boy two years earlier from his sister, who had in turn obtained the boy from an orphanage.

"Pseudo" child abuse may be presented to medical and psychiatric facilities. These involve the use of various folk treatments, such as moxybustion, "coining," acupuncture, and deep kneading or pounding. Instances of lead and arsenic poisoning from administration of folk medications have also occurred among refugee children (Kerr and Saryan, 1986); these may cause permanent brain damage. Although these folk methods have actually been recommended for refugee children by the United Nations High Commission for Refugees, they can and do involve certain complications. For example, acupuncture with unclean needles has caused hepatitis B, and refugee children have been subject to brain damage from lead-containing folk nostrums. Refugee parents should be instructed to avoid medically unsupervised oral administration of drugs and treatments that break the skin of their children.

Racism and Harassment. These untoward experiences are not anticipated by many refugees who come from communities in which they comprised the dominant race or culture (while this is not true for refugees who formerly belonged to minorities, such as ethnic Chinese from Indochina and Soviet Jews from the U.S.S.R.). Even in camps, refugees tend to be placed with others of the same culture. With resettlement to the United States, the reality of minority status takes hold. Especially in lower-class neighborhoods, indigenous American neighbors typically resent refugees' competition for unskilled jobs, low-cost housing, and finite health and social services. Hostility may spill over into vandalism, harassment, assault, and other forms of persecution. Some racial hostility can occur among diverse refugee groups, whose hostilities may predate their arrival in the United States. Refugee children may become the victims of hostile attitudes, as well as the perpetrators through their acting out of parental or community hostility.

Case 4: An 18-year-old Vietnamese man was referred by the court for evaluation after having stabbed another student, a Lao refugee. He assaulted the fellow student after being repeatedly harassed on ethnic grounds. He was perpetuating a pattern of behavior that he had adopted only recently in the refugee camp, and that was supported by his family and peers. Recommendations to the court and school included the following: (1) challenging the young man's notions of problem-solving as being unacceptable in this country, (2) a period of probation and counseling regarding alternate methods of problem-solving, and (3) revocation of probation if assaults recurred. There were no subsequent assaults.

Identity conflicts. Such conflicts occur among refugee children and adolescents who are, like their indigenous American peers, in the process of developing an individual sense of self. For refugee children, the process is complicated by the fact that the majority society and their peers at school are "Americanizing" them in one fashion while their parents and expatriate communities are ensocializing them in another fashion. This situation resembles that described for other cultural minorities in the United States (Katz, 1979; Levy, 1933). Most refugee children cope with bicultural adaptation reasonably well (Szapocznik, Kurtines, and Fernandez, 1980), but some vulnerable children do not (Naditch and Morrissey, 1976). As Leichty (1963) observed in her study of Vietnamese children in Vietnam and American children in the United States, aged 9 to 11 years, cultures can produce markedly dissimilar self-concept and attitudes toward family, others, and society at large. Children and adolescents isolated from refugee peers may have particular difficulties with this task due to the absence of peers facing like developmental tasks. In children thus deprived of mutual vicarious learning, problems may arise, as in this case.

Case 5: A 15-year-old Hmong girl, the eldest in her family, lived with her family in a remote rural community, where the nearest Hmong family was over 2 hours away by car. Her parents had forbidden her to socialize with American peers. She came for medical attention with numerous somatic symptoms and symptoms of minor anxiety and depression, leading to numerous school absences and then to subsequent academic failure. In addition to rage with her parents, she had poor self-esteem. Intervention consisted of biweekly supportive visits and the recommendation to her family that they move closer to other Hmong families. Her parents followed this recommendation at the end of the school year, leading to resolution of her symptoms within several weeks. Over this time she was able to befriend other Hmong adolescents in her same situation, while learning ways of coping with both her family, the larger society, and her interest in socializing with age mates.

Refugee adolescents may reject their traditional culture and "go native." Many of them readily adopt local teenage grooming, clothes, behaviors, and expressions (i.e., superficial aspects of American society). This may occur without acquiring education and skills to succeed in this highly competitive society (Tobin and Friedman, 1984). At times this "going native" is associated with parent-child conflict.

Failure to Acculturate. Failure to acculturate often precipitates problems in refugee families. Like their parents and grandparents, refugee children and adolescents are also engaged in adjusting to a new society. This process requires adapting to new language, modes of nonverbal communication, clothes, climate, topography, diet, values, customs, and etiquette. Most refugee youth accomplish these tasks more easily and completely than do their elders. This enhanced ability to adapt of youth does not diminish the difficulty and stress imposed by this adaptive task, however. This youthful ability can be undermined by one or more of several factors.

— Brain impairment, so that new knowledge and skills are not acquired

— Isolation in an expatriate community, so that access to the majority society is not available to refugee youth

— Shyness from risk-taking and episodic failure experiences

Family Problems

Refugee families may precipitate or exacerbate problems in their children. Likewise, refugee family members are often key actors in the amelioration of their children's discomforts, disabilities, and maladjustments. Refugee families are undergoing changes and stresses unlike those of local families; these are reviewed here. The clinician must bear in mind that refugee families can have difficulties similar to those of American families (e.g., divorce, incest).

Role Reversal. Role reversal can occur due to more rapid acculturation among refugee children, as compared to the parents, causing refugee children to assume adult roles. These roles and activities may be relatively benign, such as the child's translating for the parent at a grocery store. However, these responsibilities often expand to include children's screening phone calls and visitors, translating confidential medical interviews, or managing the family budget. Preteen or teenage children may dominate or attempt to dominate the family. Resultant problems can vary from the child's being deprived of an ordinary childhood to the child's domination and even physical abuse of parents or grandparents.

Partial Families and Solo Parents. These family structures are common in some refugee groups, due to death of one or both parents, incarceration of a parent in the homeland, or disagreement within families regarding flight (so that only part of a family flees). Since men are more apt to have died in military action or to have been imprisoned for political reasons, the solo parent is most likely to be a woman. For example, 23 percent of 37,844 Vietnamese households in the United States were headed by a woman in 1976 (Kelly, 1977). Conflict may intrude when adolescent sons believe that they should dominate their solo-parent mothers. Difficulties in solo-father families are usually due to inadequate parenting skills or involvement rather than inadequate parental authority. Some children in partial families may be supervised only at school, and allowed to roam on their own at other times.

Case 6: A 14-year-old Vietnamese boy was referred by the school for drug use at school and disruptive behavior in the classroom. Both his parents and his two siblings had died during escape. Two single male cousins in their twenties had legal custody for the boy. Former soldiers who were uneducated and unskilled, the cousins were engaged in episodic unskilled labor, petty crime, gambling, and drug sales. Foster placement was arranged, along with therapy for missed bereavement. The boy's behavioral problems at school cleared uneventfully.

Changing Sex Roles. In many (but not all) Third World countries, the daily work and activities of men and women differ greatly. For example, in many areas of Southeast Asia, farmers and tribal women haul water, gather firewood, bear and care for the children, clean and decorate the household, make and repair clothes, cultivate the garden, tend small animals, and prepare and cook food. Men farm or fish, tend large animals, build the house, hunt, help with local community projects (e.g., repair roads or bridges), and engage in various semiskilled tasks (e.g., carpentry, boat-making). Literally, men and women need one another to survive since no one man or woman has adequate skills or time to perform all the chores necessary to survive. These traditional sex role differences may later present problems for refugee children, since the traditional parental role models may not be relevant to adult roles as they will encounter them in their future lives (Westermeyer, Bouafuely, and Vang, 1984).

Intergenerational Conflict. This type of conflict often ensues as the children acculturate more rapidly than their parents and grandparents. It varies in duration and intensity, and in its effects on parents and children. Adolescence is a vulnerable phase as refugee minors are trying to establish their own identities, court, and enter mainstream social recreation and work roles. Dating and marriage are often focal issues. Tragedies may result. For example, a Hmong father hanged himself when his son, without the father's permission, bought a new car with money that the son himself had earned.

Parental Acculturation Failure. Refugee parents who fail to learn English, to understand American social institutions, or to enter the world of work are less effective in preparing their children for life in the United States than those who do. Parental liabilities range from inability to cooperate with the school system in the education of their children, to inability to serve as role models or to teach relevant social survival skills to their children. In addition, such nonacculturating parents put themselves at risk to crises precipitated by unfamiliar behavior among their acculturating children, as in the following case.

Case 7: A Hmong family was referred from the emergency room after the mother had attempted suicide by swallowing pills. The family crisis was precipitated unknowingly by their eldest 14-year-old daughter, who had allowed a 14-year-old Hmong boy to carry her books home from school. When she introduced the boy to her mother at the door, her mother began weeping, tearing at her clothes, and later ingested pills. The mother assumed that the girl had become sexually active and was trying to force a marriage on her parents (neither of which was the case). Following resolution of the family crisis (and during treatment for associated psychiatric and medical problems in the parents), the parents were introduced to a local sign language class. They learned rapidly, and the family reintegrated on a more stable and acculturated level.

Parental Psychiatric Disorder. Major depression, substance abuse, schizophrenia, or other disorder in parents can result in their being unable to discharge parental responsibilities effectively, putting their children at risk of subsequent personality, interpersonal, and mental-emotional problems. Studies of refugee parents from World War II have indicated that even less serious but long-lasting parental traits may adversely affect children, for example, a lingering distrust of the outside world (Freyberg, 1980); the imposition on their children of a duty to compensate them for their own earlier losses (Trossman, 1968); or the assignment of names and roles to children who are expected to replace the lost relatives for whom they were named (Rakoff, 1964). Even so-called invulnerable children may evolve out of this process with social competence, but with poor interpersonal skills and with problems caring for themselves emotionally (Anthony and Cohler, 1987).

Family Structure and Adaptive Style. Like individuals, refugee families bring their own structures, functions, and histories (Dunnigan, 1982). These may foster individual and family adaptation in the United States, or they may impede it. Structures and styles that were successful in the former culture may be problem-producing in the United States if they are continued rigidly without respect for changed circumstances. Economic pursuits, recreation, age and sex roles, courting and marriage practices, childbearing, and child raising occur within the context of the family. To the extent that the family can support its members as they undergo changes in these areas, the family aids adjustment. To the extent that the family impedes such changes, it may add to its children's burdens.

Case 8: A 17-year-old Cambodian refugee had done extremely well in high school, to the point of taking mostly college courses in his last year of school. Whenever not studying, however, he was plagued with migraine headaches. Although socially skilled and pleasant, he had no friends. His father and eldest brother had been murdered in Cambodia, and his second eldest brother had recently married and (in the patient's eyes) "deserted" the family for California. This left the patient as the eldest male in the home with his mother and four younger siblings. Treatment involved helping him deal with the family deaths (which he had not grieved) and his rage at his second eldest brother for leaving the family. In a family session, his mother expressed her hope that he would continue college; this greatly relieved and supported him. His migraines abated after a few sessions. After several sessions, he was befriending both American and Cambodian students and was allowing time for leisure and social activities.

Psychopathology

Symptom Levels Among Refugee Children. A study of 96 Thai Dam (from Laos) and Vietnamese students in grades 7 to 10 was conducted using self-assessment rating scales. Findings indicated a lower perceived adaptation to school in the United States 4 years after resettlement as compared to perceived adaptation to school in Asia. Refugee students also reported lower grades in the United States as compared to Asia. Younger students and students with higher grades in English tended to have a self-perception of better adaptation to the United States (Nguyen and Henkin, 1980), as compared to older students and those with lower English grades.

Krupinski and Burrows and co-workers (1986) have studied Indochinese children and adolescents in Australia, using reports from children, parents, and teachers in addition to selected psychiatric interviewing. Results showed high symptom levels in the months following arrival, notably greater than those of indigenous Australian children. On follow-up of only a nonrandom part of this group, the Indochinese children were much improved. However, the high dropout rate in this follow-up study (too high to allow conclusions) make the data suspect.

Charron and Ness (1977) studied 67 Vietnamese adolescents in Connecticut aged 13 to 19 years using the Cornell Medical Index (CMI). The mean CMI score for this group was twice as high as that reported for a group of Vietnamese adults in Seattle. (This comparative finding of Vietnamese adolescents versus adults is difficult to interpret, since American adolescents also report higher symptom levels than American adults on many self-rating scales and certain scales of psychological tests, such as the Minnesota Multiphasic Personality Inventory.) Higher symptom levels were reported by refugee Vietnamese adolescents who had more frequent arguments with parents ($r = 0.37$), less part-time employment ($r = -0.33$); and fewer American friends ($r = -0.38$)— findings similar to those of Krupinski and Burrows (1986). A greater number of years of education in the United States showed up as significantly associated with lower symptom levels on a stepwise multiple regression.

Morgan, Wingard, and Felice (1984) administered anonymous questionnaires on alcohol use to 69 Indochinese aged 16 to 22 years at the San Diego Job Care Center. As compared to white, black, and Hispanic youth, fewer Indochinese used alcohol regularly (i.e., 44 of 69). However, the Indochinese drinkers were most apt to state that they drank to forget (59 percent vs. 21 percent to 47 percent for the other groups). These Indochinese youths—who had been residents of the United States for only about 1 year—also reported lower levels of vocational, legal, or medical problems associated with drinking as compared to the other three groups.

Special Vulnerability. Sack et al. (1986) compared 40 Cambodian adolescents who survived the Pol Pot horrors with 6 Cambodian adolescents who had fled their homeland prior to that time. Most of the students were in grades 10 and 11. Despite the small numbers, Pol Pot survivors were significantly more apt to receive a psychiatric diagnosis based on a thorough assessment. Teachers rated more Pol Pot survivors as "deviant" on two or more behavioral items, and as more emotionally withdrawn. However, academic achievement and disciplinary incidents in school did not vary between the groups.

Organic Brain Syndromes, Organic Personality Disorder, Organic Affective Disorder, and Organic Mental Disorder. Inadequate parental care, infection, malnutrition, trauma, and vehicular accidents are common causes for these disorders among refugee children. Later onset in childhood often alters the typical clinical picture observed in American children. These later acquired cases of brain damage may not appear as dysfunctional as the birth-onset or constitutional cases. Those with acquired organic disorders may retain trite social skills, the ability to read, and greater vocabulary, while being impaired in their ability to learn new materials and solve new problems. Organic brain damage can also influence personality and social development, leaving children at risk to subsequent maladjustment and psychiatric disorder.

Case 9: A 15-year-old Lao male high school student was seen with an acute psychosis. At age 10 he had a high sustained fever in a refugee camp, with febrile convulsions and two days of coma. Subsequently, he showed a personality change with greater impulsiveness, irritability, self-centeredness, and problems with authority. During his preteen and early adolescent years he experienced mounting problems in coping with peer relationships, authority figures, and sexuality, although he continued to achieve A grades in school until shortly before his mental illness.

Learning Disabilities. These disabilities are difficult to assess in recently arrived refugee children. However, these disorders should be considered in refugee children who do poor academic work or fail over time to learn English on a level with peers. Attention deficit hyperactivity disorder may also undermine academic progress and social adjustment. Medical, neurological, and psychiatric evaluation along with culture-fair psychological testing should be undertaken in such cases, since the usual English psychometric measures have dubious validity in children whose primary language is not English. Neurological signs, history of central nervous system damage, and psychiatric evaluation can lead to remedial recommendations to family, school, or other social resources.

Mental Retardation. Adjustment problems can ensue in retarded refugee children who previously achieved social and behavioral stability in the country of origin. With supervision and direction, most of them had previously assumed family roles and delimited work responsibilities. Refugee flight to a nearby country or relocation to the United States can disrupt this stability, leading to behavioral, emotional, or mental disorders. Family stability and role continuity are important in preventing morbidity in this group.

Case 10: A 14-year-old Hmong boy with moderate mental retardation was presented in the emergency department after assaulting family members. Examination revealed paranoid hallucinations and delusions. Previously he had gotten along well in the family. During the family's recent flight out of Laos, the father—a local chief—died when he stepped on a land mine while leading the village. Since arrival in the United States, the patient's mother and three older siblings had been out of the home regularly with school and English language courses. After having been arrested for meandering through traffic, the patient had been locked up alone in the apartment (he previously had always been with relatives 24 hours a day). Next he left water running and burned himself on the gas stove, resulting in his being locked alone in his room for long periods when family members were not present at home. Following a period of hospitalization and neuroleptic medication, he did well in a day program for moderately retarded adolescents, supplemented by family counseling.

Major Depression. The most common psychiatric disorder among refugee adults (Westermeyer, 1988, 1989), major depression is also frequent among refugee teenagers aged 16 years or older who come to clinical attention. Refugee preteenagers and early teenagers are diagnosed infrequently as having a major depression. This latter finding may be due to the low prevalence of major depression among children and younger teens generally, as compared to older teens and adults. It may also be due to the difficulty of recognizing depression in children, with its somewhat different manifestations (e.g., hypersomnia rather than insomnia, social conflict rather than social withdrawal, aggressiveness rather than self-punitiveness) and its variable presentation with the child's age (Ionescu-Tongyonk, 1977; Philips, 1979; Welner, 1978). Depressive symptoms in refugee children and adolescents often accompany other problems that impede adjustment, such as learning, conduct, or substance use disorders. These associated conditions can also make it difficult to recognize the separate existence of major depression.

Case 11: A 10-year-old Hmong orphan manifested numerous symptoms after her mother's death; for example, nightmares, night terrors, fear of being alone, fear of flushing toilets, aversion to bathing, an exaggerated need to please adults, inability to reveal anger toward adults, with episodic rages against her siblings, stealing from mother surrogates and envied peers who still had both parents, and lying to cover her stealing and to avoid any displeasure from adults. After a year in a foster family setting, the first five symptoms disappeared whereas the others persisted (albeit at a lower rate). On psychiatric evaluation, she revealed the idea that her misbehavior had caused her mother to die, and the fear that adults would abandon her if she expressed anger. She manifested a profound depressed mood with prolonged weeping—something she had hidden from adults and peers for fear that it would alienate them. When several psychotherapy sessions failed to alleviate her profound depression, imipramine was begun and increased to therapeutic blood levels (this required 150 mg). She improved considerably during 9 months of weekly psychotherapy, permitting gradual discontinuation of medication.

Mania. Like depression, mania can be difficult to recognize in adolescents even within American society (Ballenger, Reus, and Post, 1982). Early on, cases may be misidentified as schizophrenia, conduct disorder, attention deficit-hyperactivity disorder, or other diagnoses. Across cultural and language boundaries, in a context of refugee migration, the classic mania picture can be even more modified and difficult to appreciate. Alienation, failure to acculturate, antiauthority stances, inappropriate sexuality, and other attitudinal-behavior problems may dominate the picture. Psychological symptoms are present (e.g., racing thoughts, grandiosity, simple hallucinations), but must be inquired after since they are rarely volunteered. Classic adult vegetative symptoms (e.g., hyposomnia, weight loss) may be absent in adolescents. Lapses in judgment or fluctuations in attention may be hard to identify since normal adolescents may episodically manifest similar lapses and fluctuations (although for brief rather than prolonged periods). To a large extent, the key to this diagnosis lies in first considering it, and then establishing whether the disorder is present. Therapeutic trials may be needed to confirm the diagnosis.

Case 12: A 17-year-old unaccompanied Vietnamese boy was referred due to irascibility, argumentativeness, alienation from peers, failure to respond to limit setting, and academic failure. Over the previous year his behavior had led to expulsion from three schools and from four foster families; during this time he had been treated three times a week by a psychoanalyst. Assessment revealed grandiose delusions, racing thoughts, flight of ideas, and simple hallucinations. Lithium reduced most of the patient's severely disruptive behavior within several days, so that he was able to return to school. Subsequently he was able to remain with the same family, finish high school, and continue on to college.

Schizophrenia, Schizophreniform, and Paranoid Psychosis. These conditions often appear in young refugees who are vulnerable as a result of preexisting brain insult. Refugee families typically have difficulty accepting the gravity and chronicity of the problem. This lack of acceptance can have untoward consequences for the patient, other family members, and the family finances. Families often engage in recurrent help-seeking at a variety of medical, social and psychiatric facilities, undermining long-term rehabilitative efforts. Families may expend large sums on folk healing modalities, which can offer temporary hope but rarely affect the long-term course. Some families may resist seeking help, especially if the affected adolescent is docile and withdrawn.

When a new refugee group arrives in the United States, they typically bring few schizophrenics or other chronically mentally ill persons with them. Mentally ill persons have either been left behind or have not survived the flight. Thus, the need for services to such persons is initially very low. Over time, however, the need increases as new cases appear. The prevalence rate of these disorders among refugees and other migrants significantly exceeds their rate in the general American population (Westermeyer, 1989), probably due both to prearrival victimizations and brain insults as well as postarrival acculturation stresses. Thus, long-term program planning must take into account the need for specialized services to this group.

Psychoactive Substance Use Disorders. These disorders have been reported in numerous refugee groups (Westermeyer, 1989). Initially after resettlement the prevalence of substance abuse is low to nil (Morgan, Wingard, and Felice, 1984). As time goes on, the extent of the problem increases in refugees of all age groups, including the youth.

Case 13: A 15-year-old Hmong orphan was brought to psychiatric assessment by his uncle for school failure and social withdrawal at home; marijuana smoking was suspected. The patient's parents and three siblings had all been shot in the Mekong River while attempting to flee Laos. Soon after, at age 12, he had begun smoking cannabis in the refugee camp. This behavior persisted in the United States, where he had joined other minority youth selling cannabis to fellow students. Urine was positive for cannabis.

Case 14: A 17-year-old unaccompanied Cuban girl from the Mariel flight was referred by the court after having been arrested with her 38-year-old Cuban boyfriend for dealing cocaine. The girl was found to have cocaine dependence and met criteria for a conduct disorder.

Eating Disorders. Obesity is the usual eating problem observed among refugees of all ages, especially when they have been food-deprived. Anorexia and bulimia are not yet common problems among refugee adolescents. Nonetheless, occasional cases of the latter conditions are reported as refugees become more influenced by their American peers.

Case 15: A 17-year-old Lao girl was evaluated for overeating, weight loss, and amenorrhea. She admitted to recently initiating bulimia, a practice that she had learned from American friends. Treatment with this well-acculturated, intelligent patient was standard, supplemented with culturally sensitive family therapy.

Conduct Disorders. These adolescent disorders are associated with various past and current victimization, psychiatric conditions, and family problems. Their diversity defies any simple classification. Numerous case vignettes in this report provide examples. The following case exemplifies the past and current stressors often present in these cases.

A 12-year-old Lao boy was evaluated for touching girls' genitalia in class, assault on other children, and failure to respond to teachers' limit setting. History revealed that the boy's father, a former policeman, had become mentally ill and gone to live in a Buddhist temple after the Communist regime was established. Subsequently, his mother began a liaison with a Vietnamese soldier who eventually moved in and forced the patient and his elder teenage brothers out of the home. The brothers brought the boy to a refugee camp in Thailand and then returned to fight with the resistance in Laos. As an unaccompanied minor, the boy was placed with an American woman with a long history of recurrent mental illness. One of the woman's teenage sons alerted authorities that his mother was deteriorating again and that she had been appearing partially clothed in the home, leaving the bathroom door open while she bathed, and fondling the children in a seductive fashion. The boy responded to placement with a Lao family and psychotherapy over a one-year period.

Post-traumatic Stress Disorder (PTSD). Terr (1981) showed that children demonstrate post-traumatic symptoms for months following a psychologically traumatic event. In her study of the Chowchilla school bus kidnap victims, she found that all victimized children developed symptoms of variable nature, severity, and duration. These included displaced fears, fear of subsequent threat, repeated dreams or nightmares, reenactment of the event, personality change, misperceptions, overgeneralizations, and time distortion. Krupinski, Burrows, and co-workers (1986) have also reported high symptom levels among children and adolescents in the early months following resettlement in Australia.

Parental Somatization of Refugee Children. Although parental somatization is not a formal psychiatric diagnosis, it nonetheless occurs frequently enough to warrant special attention. Refugee parents may bring normal children to medical attention due to displacement of their own parental anxiety onto their children. Medical reassurance fails to alleviate this repeated, expensive, unhelpful, and misdirected behavior. Psychiatric assessment of the parent is warranted. Pediatricians, family physicians, public health nurses, and social workers should be aware of this common problem by which refugee parents call attention to themselves and their families.

Case 16: An 8-year-old Hmong child was brought to psychiatric attention after the father had repeatedly brought the child to numerous dental, pediatric, and hospital clinics. He complained of an abnormality of his child's tongue (lymphatic tissue on the tongue, a normal benign variant). He ascribed numerous "misbehaviors" to this malady; these consisted of essentially normal "American child" behaviors that his daughter had learned in school and from peers. We agreed to assess his child psychologically if the father allowed us to assess him. He agreed and was found to have a major depression. The child's testing revealed her to be a normal, comfortable child with superior intelligence, who was functioning well in school.

Failure to Thrive. This condition, also not a formal diagnosis, is apt to occur in refugee families overwhelmed by losses, stresses, and new adjustments.

Case 17: A young Lao couple brought their emaciated 9-month-old child to medical attention. Their first-born child had died in a refugee camp shortly before the birth of this child. Hospitalized for assessment, this second infant ate voraciously and was soon approaching normal weight. The family interview revealed that the maternal grandmother had declared the infant a "spirit baby"—that is, the reincarnation of the dead child, come back to die again and thus cause further misery to the parents. In family therapy the parents were guided in grieving their earlier loss—a process that they had not undergone in the midst of this infant's birth and the transition from camp to the United States. Further, it was suggested that the child's rapid growth in the hospital indicated that the child was not a "spirit baby." The grandmother changed her assessment of the child. The child's subsequent course was very good.

Delayed Disorders. These have been described in people who were refugees as children by Krell (1985a, 1985b, 1988). Psychiatric disorders with trauma-related content have occurred decades later in those who were Holocaust survivors or Japanese concentration camp internees as children. These disorders were precipitated decades later by various environmental events. Krell's methods of dealing with these resemble therapy for PTSD. Such problems occurring years or even decades later—in association with retirement, death of a spouse, a robbery, vandalism, assault, or loss of a job—are also common among those who were adults at the time of refugee flight, and thus are not specific to refugee children alone.

Data Collection

Assessment of refugee minors follows the same principles as assessment of other youth, with certain modifications. As with adults, the examiner ascertains the nature of the current problem, medical history, family illnesses, and social background, along with a physical examination and screening laboratory tests. Developmental data must be obtained, including prenatal, natal, and postnatal health problems; progression of the child's behavioral and psychosocial development; and current developmental status. This must include both cultural development within the culture of origin as well as acculturation to the new society (Westermeyer, 1985, 1987a,b). Family assessment, important for adults, is critical for children and adolescents. Only special aspects of refugee assessment are covered here, but the routine data sought for young indigenous patients should be obtained.

Refugee Flight Story. As with adults, it is important to inquire specifically regarding the events associated with the refugee flight. These include preflight stressors, rationales for flight, dangers and losses along the way, conditions in the refugee camp and duration of time spent there, and conditions of the early resettlement in the United States. Family status before, during, and after the flight should be ascertained. Age at leaving the culture of origin and upon arriving in the United States should be determined.

History of Violence and Threat. In many regions undergoing conflict, refugee children have been beaten, tortured, and murdered. They may also be wounded in the midst of hostilities. Routine inquiry must be made regarding this, since the child or parents may not reveal such events spontaneously.

Developmental Status vis-à-vis Culture. Culture has little influence on early neuromotor and psychosocial development, including such development hallmarks as sitting, walking, talking, and climbing. In cultures where adults more or less constantly carry, hold, or attend the child, unusually early toilet training may be reported—although it is probably the parents who are "trained" to anticipate the children's signals of impending urination and defecation. Later in childhood and adolescence numerous indices of development can be heavily influenced by culture. These include attaining literacy, courting, assuming adult responsibilities, and achieving independent decision-making. In some societies an individual is not viewed as a mature, independent adult until his or her grandchildren are born. Predictably, the age at flight and relocation greatly influence cultural aspects of psychosocial development. The case described earlier in which a Hmong father committed suicide when his son decided on his own to buy a car exemplifies the son's lack of appreciation of his father's concept of adult status, and the father's lack of understanding regarding the son's new cultural norms for adult status. Kremer and Sabin (1985) have identified similar problems based on their work with 21 Indochinese refugee children and adolescents.

Working with a Translator. Recently arrived refugees or those who have not acquired adequate English must be assessed with the aid of a translator (unless the clinician speaks the patient's native language). In the clinical context, translators are often referred to as interpreters (since it is to be hoped that they will convey connotative as well as denotative meaning) or bilingual workers (since their responsibilities generally involve much more than translation or interpretation).

The patient-interpreter relationship can be different when the patient is a child rather than an adult. The child's transference to the interpreter may involve distrust, fear of being judged, or loss of confidentiality through the interpreter to the parents. Or conversely, due to the presence of an interpreter, the child may trust the "foreign" clinician who is teamed up with a person from the child's own ethnic group.

Similarly the interpreter's "countertransference" can affect the interview with the child. An interpreter may react negatively to the child's acculturation or Americanization, or an interpreter may preach to or shame a refugee minor who needs understanding and support. Conversely, the interpreter may seek to establish a therapeutic alliance with the child. The clinician-interpreter relationship also can be crucial in this process. Interpreters or clinicians unprepared for this complex task may not be fit for it (Hoang and Erickson, 1985).

Family Assessment. Meeting, interviewing, and assessing the family is as important for refugee children as for other children. However, it often requires longer sessions and more visits in order to establish rapport and mutual trust, and to clear up misunderstandings that commonly occur on both sides. If a translator must be used, this can also retard the process, adding to the time and expense. Experienced bilingual workers can often facilitate the process by meeting briefly with the family first without the clinician, and then later with the clinician. Especially if a rigid matriarch or patriarch is domineering or obstructing the interviews, separate interviews with individual family members may also be fruitful. If an extended family is involved, an interview with them can aid in clarifying family dynamics; these interviews usually require a few hours (Spiegel, 1982).

Psychological Testing. Psychiatrists, pediatricians, and neurologists rely heavily on psychologists for quantification or specification of certain conditions. Development of psychological testing norms in the United States are based on the assumption that children have been exposed to English from birth and to the American educational system. To the extent that these assumptions are not true, testing can be erroneous—especially if administered or interpreted in a rigid "cookbook" fashion. Like the cross-cultural nurse, psychiatrist, or social worker, the cross-cultural psychologist must thoroughly appreciate the dimensions of the function being evaluated, means for accomplishing that task, and test bias introduced by illiteracy or inability to speak English. Skill and experience in interpreting the test results are crucial. Knowledge and supervision by culturally sensitive mentors are key elements in preparing competent psychologists for cross-cultural work (Williams, 1985).

Validity and Reliability. In the psychiatric evaluation of adults, much (but by no means all) data originate from the patient's anamnesis and the clinician's observations. This is inadequate for assessment of most children. Extensive information must ordinarily be obtained from parents and teachers. In some cases data are also obtained from other relatives, social workers, public health nurses, police, courts, and other physicians.

In a study of Cambodian children who survived the Pol Pot horrors, Sack et al. (1986) found that most parents underestimated their children's psychological and social difficulties, as compared to the children's assessments of themselves and their teachers' assessments. Krupinski, Burrows, and co-workers (1986) made a similar observation among Indochinese children and adolescents in Australia; most families were Vietnamese. This same trend for parents to under-report their children's problems has been observed in a study of American children and their parents (Weissman et al., 1987). Thus, this finding is not a refugee-specific one.

Even such matters as the patient's age may have variable cultural validity. For example, Vietnamese and ethnic Chinese children may be assumed to be one year at the time of birth as a result of one year in utero. Families may underestimate a child's age to gain more years in the school system (due to lost years before or after flight). Or a child's age may be exaggerated to gain early access to the labor market, so family finances can be enhanced. In these latter cases reliability may be good, but validity is poor. It may be necessary to obtain bone age if an objective approximation in age is needed.

TREATMENT

Model Program

Treatment of refugee children and adolescents closely resembles that of indigenous youth in one sense: the choice of a particular modality is based on diagnosis, dynamic assessment, and context. Therapeutic modalities are not uniquely culture-bound. The application of these modalities is related to cultural factors, however. As with other children and adolescents, a continuum of culturally sensitive psychiatric services are necessary for refugee youth (McKelvey, 1988).

Three aspects of a model psychiatric program for refugee children have been described so far. One of these is the hiring and training of refugees to serve as translators, interpreters, outreach and follow-up workers, educators, and social supports for refugee families with disturbed or disturbing members. Second, staff members in various disciplines must be trained to discharge their clinical responsibilities in a culturally sensitive way. Third, adequate care for refugees requires extra time, which must be reflected in adequate staff/patient ratios. Other characteristics of a model refugee program for children include the following.

— Access to psychometric and radiographic assessment of brain impairment

— Liaison and outreach with schools, courts, resettlement agencies, and pediatric and family practice clinics

— Availability of programs for refugee children with special training and educational needs, including mental retardation, borderline intelligence, learning disabilities, and attention deficit disorder

— Awareness regarding high vulnerability among refugee children at special risk (e.g., children in solo-parent or other partial families, children of parents with substance abuse or other chronic or recurrent psychopathology, Pol Pot survivors and other victims, children with brain injuries, unaccompanied minors, and mixed-race Amerasian children)

— Stable funding that will persist over decades, since the need persists over time

— Development of cross-cultural expertise among staff members through subsidized training, conferences, speakers, consultants, journals, books, and videotapes

All therapeutic modalities must be administered in a culturally sensitive way. This includes not only counseling and psychodynamically oriented psychotherapy, but also behavior modification, pharmacotherapy, and other somatotherapies. Characteristics of culturally sensitive treatment that have been described (Ananth, 1984; Hoang and Erickson, 1985; Lee, 1988; Szapocznik et al., 1978; Westermeyer, 1989) include the following.

— The clinician should have some general awareness of the patient's cultural values, attitudes, ideal-versus-behavioral norms, and world view.

— More specific cultural knowledge must be obtained relative to the particular symptoms, conflicts, problems, or context presented by the patient (e.g., social activities that are socially approved for solo parents, age at initiating courting in an adolescent, relative value accorded to independence from family versus family interdependence for older adolescents).

— The clinician should appreciate the major stressors acting on the young, minority, acculturating patient and be able to recognize the strengths and resources available to the young refugee patient in his or her sociocultural situation (Hill, 1975).

— The patient's concepts of health, illness, well-being, and disease should be known by the therapist. It is often useful to ask refugee youth about their ideas regarding the cause of the problem, its probable course, and possible outcomes.

Pharmacotherapy

Some pharmacodynamic and pharmacokinetic data do exist for adults from various racial and ethnic groups. These indicate that, at a fixed dose of tricyclic, whites have lower blood levels than Asians, Asian-Americans, and Afro-Americans (Allen, Rack, and Vaddadi, 1977; Lewis et al., 1980; Ziegler and Biggs, 1977). Whites also maintain lower blood levels of neuroleptics at a fixed dose (Patkin et al., 1984; Young, 1983). Pharmacokinetics of lithium do not appear to vary across races, although psychiatrists in Asia achieve clinical response at blood levels below those employed in the United States (Okuma, 1981; Yang, 1985). All of these studies involve adults. Unfortunately, such studies across cultures and races do not yet exist for children. If these data are extrapolated to children, lower doses of tricyclics, neuroleptics, and even possibly lithium may be effective for refugee children who are not white. However, the interpatient differences greatly exceed the inter-racial or interethnic differences, so the psychiatrist must individualize the dose and not shy away from employing adequate doses.

Compliance problems and complaints regarding side effects may occur more often among refugee patients, who are frequently not familiar with taking long-term medications or medications that cause bothersome side effects. These can be reduced by careful education and reeducation of the parents and the child. Routine instructions include the following.

— The medication must not be given to siblings, relatives, or friends. Refugees unfamiliar with psychotropic agents may share prescription drugs or "prescribe" them for others with like symptoms.

— Higher doses must not be taken without physician approval. Some Third World people, mainly experienced with drugs such as penicillin, believe that if a little is good then more must be better.

— Most psychotropic medications require weeks to show their first effects, and they may need to be taken for months or even years. Many refugees have a model of pharmacotherapy derived from aspirin or penicillin, and so expect relief in hours or a few days, with cessation of need for medication in several hours or days.

— The prescribing physician must know all other medications being taken, including other prescribed drugs, over-the-counter drugs, folk remedies, and illicit drugs such as opium. Not to do so can undermine the efficacy of psychotropic medication, perhaps make matters worse, or possibly prove fatal. Faced with severe or disabling illness, some Third World refugees "doctor shop" without informing the respective physicians. Over-the-counter and herbal drugs often have antihistaminic, anticholinergic, sedative, or sympathomimetic effects. Abuse of opium, alcohol, cannabis, and other drugs retards recovery; these substances may also counteract or potentiate side effects or complications of psychotropic medication.

— Medication alone rarely solves psychiatric problems. On the physician's part, there is usually need for counsel, direction, suggestion, education, recommendations, or psychotherapy. On the patient's part, there is usually need for redirection, change, effort, or forbearance. Refugees and their families may expect that a pill might magically change psychopathology without any other efforts being expended, especially if they conceive of their illness as being solely biomedical—a common notion among somatizing refugees.

Education, Counseling, and Therapy

One hears the opinion that Third World people cannot be treated with psychotherapy in individual, family, or group settings. It can be done, but this prevalent misconception does reflect the special problems that therapy across cultures can present. Among these are the following.

— The flow, pace, and mode of participation characteristic of therapy makes the use of a translator unwieldy. In the therapy of groups, leaders should speak the participant's language if at all possible.

— If the therapist has an ethnicity different from the group, he or she may feel overwhelmed or outnumbered, especially if inexperienced with the refugee group or insecure about such an effort.

— Family structure in the particular culture must be understood in order to develop rapport with the family and to avoid "cultural resistances" (Kim, 1985).

— A key step in being aware of others' cultures lies in first being aware of one's own culture, its implicit and often subconscious values, prescriptions, strictures, obligations, and standards (Moffic et al., 1987).

— The therapist must demonstrate respect for the familiy's or group's culture and avoid stereotyping (Lappin, 1983).

— The therapist at times acts as a "culture broker" or "change agent" to aid refugees in adapting effectively to the stressors and opportunities that impinge on their daily lives (Lappin and Scott, 1982).

— Special elements of family structure and function that should be appreciated include marriage forms and structure, family roles, mutual obligations, and family shame (Kim, 1985; Shon and Ja, 1982).

— Individual family history and value system should be discussed (McGoldrich, Pearce, and Giordano, 1982).

Rathbun, Di Virgilio, and Waldfogel (1958) first described unaccompanied refugee children, based on work with 38 refugee children brought to the United States after World War II and the Korean War. In their longitudinal survey of these children and their families, they identified clinical characteristics also seen with unaccompanied children from Asia. These latter include overeating, fear of going to sleep alone, nightmares, various phobias (e.g., fear of people), making excessive demands, overly clinging to parents, resentment of attention to siblings, repression of anger or aggression, exaggerated desire to please adults in younger children, and overt rebellion against adults in older children.

Harding and Looney (1977), working with Vietnamese refugees in a California relocation camp, noted several factors at work to dislocate unaccompanied refugee youth from refugee families that had "adopted" them as fictive family members. Camp administrators and nursing staff, who made the decision to assign "unaccompanied" status, readily permitted refugee youth to leave their "adopted" Vietnamese families and enter the separate compound for unaccompanied youth, rather than to attempt to keep the extended family unit together.

Sokoloff, Carlin, and Pham (1984) have studied 643 Vietnamese refugee children, of whom 72 percent were adopted and 20 percent were foster children (8 percent were with their own families). Common symptoms included excessive fears, jealousy, and unusual dreams; generally these abated gradually over time. Children who no longer understood Vietnamese constituted 94 percent of adopted children, 66 percent of foster children, and 0 percent of children in their own biological families. Foster and adoptive parents frequently stated that the first year after placement "drained them emotionally" due to the child's physical and emotional needs. The older children, most of whom were in foster care, had a high rate of adjustment problems similar to those of older American children in foster care. Other research on refugee and nonrefugee children from Asia has produced similar results in terms of academic achievement and psychosocial adaptation (Clark and Janisee, 1982; McBogg and Wouri, 1979).

In a study of 28 refugee adolescents, Williams and Westermeyer (1983) observed associated family problems in four of six unaccompanied refugees. In two of these families, divorced solo-parent American foster mothers (one of them mentally ill) had become overtly seductive with two adolescent males. Placement of two disturbing adolescents led to marital strife in the American families, and led to eventual separation and divorce of both foster couples. As Egan (1985) noted, assessment of these American foster families and their refugee children is a challenging but crucial task in understanding and treating these young patients. Carlin (1979) has observed that each of these children presents unique circumstances requiring individualized assessment and care.

In a recent news article on Amerasian children from Vietnam, the children were depicted as successful and adjusting well to the United

States (Lawlor, 1988). Anecdotal information from several relocation agencies is at odds with this glowing report. In one agency, 21 of 23 Amerasian refugee children required social or psychiatric services in the first year of resettlement. An occasional inter-racial refugee child still belongs to an intact family. Work with the families of these children requires what might be termed "bicultural family therapy." Jalali and Boyce (1980) have described some common features of work with these special families. The family's unresolved and divergent racial and ethnic identities remain for the child to resolve in working through to a personal and often unique identity (Faulkner and Kich, 1983).

Refugee children may reject or feel rejected by both the culture of origin and the resettlement culture and so fail to identify with or accept either society. Alienation has been described as one type of "coping mechanism" available to migratory, minority, poor, and disenfranchised youth (Lampkin, 1971). A study of Cuban refugee adolescents in Miami suggests that discontent may be in part a function of identity formation problems and role stress during acculturation (Naditch and Morrissey, 1976). Early on during resettlement, some unaccompanied adolescents have rejected both their culture of origin as well as the skill learning (e.g., acquiring the English language) needed to survive in their new society (Harding and Looney, 1977).

Health Issues

The early planning for refugees focuses on material resources and physical health: food, water, clothes, bedding, shelter, sanitation, immunization, and care of infectious disease (Stalcup et al., 1975). These emphases are important in reducing brain damage from malnutrition, exposure, and infectious disease (Westermeyer, 1987c). Important as they are, these elements are insufficient. Psychological and social needs also exist, including needs for security, play, work, education, training, interaction with peers, interaction with adults, family supervision, community boundaries and controls, formal organization, religion, and other realms. Planning, preparation, and programs in these areas are critical to child development and resettlement (or repatriation) success. Expertise in these areas is rarely in evidence. Planners, committees, and administrators typically include military and ex-military staff, former politicians, attorneys, diplomats, and other foreign service workers, whether with the Red Cross, Red Crescent, United Nations High Commission for Refugees, or various private and national organizations (Harding and Looney, 1977; Westermeyer and Williams, 1986). Arnold

(1967) has demonstrated the efficacy of early involvement of mental health experts in planning of migration, using Peace Corps workers.

Refugee parents arrive in the resettlement country with skills to raise their children in the society of origin. Many of these skills are relevant in the refugee camp or resettlement community, but others are incomplete or counterproductive in the new setting. Areas that should be covered in parental education and training include the following: nutrition, health, role stress, and culture change in refugee children family units, education, parental effectiveness, social resources in the United States, child and family law in the United States, and child raising practices in the cross-cultural context (Cone, 1979; Hill, 1975).

Refugee problems are often too extensive and complex for individual persons or families to address alone. Expatriate associations can be effective in addressing refugee problems, reinforcing a positive ethnic identity, and offering a venue for mutual support among refugees (Rumbaut and Rumbaut, 1976). Parents can meet and discuss problems, parenting experiences (e.g., privileges, limit setting) and child-related social institutions (e.g., schools, recreation programs, clinics). For children and especially adolescents, peer discussions aid in coping with the clashes among the parental culture, the peer culture, and the school culture. Expatriate groups can also contribute to refugee readjustment by providing an organization within which the individual's opinions and decisions can count, and by providing a sense of direction and control. All too often, refugees come up against organizations and programs in which nothing that they do or say has any noticeable effect—an outcome that reinforces dependency and lowers self-esteem (Seligman, 1975).

CONCLUSIONS

An adequate array of treatment and rehabilitative services for refugee youth, our future citizens, must be available. The highest priority should be given to outpatient consultation, with links to schools, clinics, and social agencies. Next, outpatient treatment should be available, with an array of somatotherapies, psychotherapies, and sociotherapies. An inpatient facility skilled in working with refugee youth is necessary for more intensive evaluation, and to deal with acute life-threatening and potentially disabling crises (e.g., suicide risk, assaultiveness, delirium), psychosis, failure of outpatient treatment, and initiation or regulation of somatotherapies. Day program or evening program care can be useful for selected cases in which the youth can function at home but not yet at school or work. Long-term residential care is necessary for a residuum of cases refractory to less intensive and extensive approaches. These cases often involve multiple problems, including various combinations of organic brain syndromes, schizophrenia, affective disorder, substance abuse, associated biomedical problems, family problems, and risks to society or to the youth.

Screening for problems of mental health and social adjustment among refugee youth should occur in several contexts. Foremost among these is the school, where a variety of academic, behavioral, and social problems are apt to be manifest. Relocation agencies and other social agencies encounter youth-related family and social problems, as do the clergy. Courts and detention centers request consultation related to violence, theft, drug dealing, and substance abuse. Primary-care clinicians and hospitals refer cases of psychosis and self-mutilation, but often miss or ignore cases of major depression, suicide risk, failure to acculturate, child abuse, incest, and persistent somatization. Staff members in all of these institutions should be sensitive to the special needs and problems of refugee youth, as well as informed about the availability of local resources and expertise.

Funding for mental health services to refugee youth is a major problem. School systems may not refer cases that they know warrant consultation because of their possible financial responsibility for costs incurred. Thus, they urge consultation through the parents, who are often not as concerned about the problem and are reluctant to spend the several hundred dollars or more often needed for a reasonably complete psychiatric assessment. Community mental health clinics in many areas do not have staff skilled in cross-cultural assessment and care and, due to inadequate funding, are reluctant to hire such staff. Health maintenance organizations (HMOs) and prepaid physician organizations (PPOs) also rarely have such staff and must obtain outside consultation—a virtual anathema since this leads to loss of revenue to outside clinics or hospitals. Refugee families with maladjusting, emotionally disturbed, or mentally ill children are more apt to be on welfare, and thus do not have access to private insurance. In order to compete with HMOs and PPOs, even private insurers in many areas are cutting back mental health benefits. Perhaps even more than the medical, social, and mental health systems, the "funding system" ("nonfunding system" would be a more accurate term) obstructs and delays adequate, timely services to refugee youth.

A major problem lies in the absence of a national policy for refugee resettlement in general, and for the mental health and social adjustment of youth in particular. Refugee youth are essentially abandoned by the federal government within months of arrival, and thrown on the not-so-tender mercies of state, county, and city government. As nonvoters and noncitizens with special and expensive needs, these future citizens do not receive services on an equitable basis. In view of their special needs, the extra time and effort required in assessment and care, and the greater level of skill required, equal care de facto means more skilled, time-consuming, and expensive care rather than simply "the same care." The lack of a national policy points up a serious weakness in the American system of government, in which the federal government may choose to pass its responsibility on to the states but the states may choose not to pick up this responsibility; the federal government then has no means to compel the states to address and pay for federal obligations. Consequently, an inhumane gap in services results for those whom our federal government has invited to this country, and who— especially in the case of refugee youth—will become our future citizens.

REFERENCES

Allen, J. J., Rack, P. H., and Vaddadi, E. S. (1977). Differences in the effects of clomipramine on English and Asian volunteers: Preliminary report on a pilot study. *Postgraduate Medical Journal, 53,* 79–86.

Ananth, J. (1984). Treatment of immigrant Indian patients. *Canadian Journal of Psychiatry, 29,* 490–493.

Anthony, E. J., and Cohler, B. J. (1987). *The Invulnerable Child.* New York: Guilford.

Arnold, C. B. (1967). Culture shock and a Peace Corps field mental health program. *Community Mental Health Journal, 3,* 53–60.

Aronson, A. M. (1984). Southeast Asian refugees in Rhode Island. *Rhode Island Medical Journal, 67,* 309.

Ballenger, J. C., Reus, V. I., and Post, R. M. (1982). The "atypical" clinical picture of adolescent mania. *American Journal of Psychiatry, 139,* 602–606.

Bogin, B., and MacVean, R. B. (1981). Biosocial effects of urban migration on the development of families and children in Guatemala. *American Journal of Public Health, 71,* 1373–1377.

Carlin, J. E. (1979). Southeast Asian refugee children. In J. D. Call, J. D. Noshpitz, R. L. Cohen, and I. N. Berlin (eds.), *Basic Handbook of Child Psychiatry,* pp. 290–300. New York: Basic Books.

Charron, D. W., and Ness, R. C. (1977). Emotional distress among Vietnamese children in a refugee camp. *American Journal of Psychiatry, 134,* 407–411.

Clark, E. A., and Janisee, J. (1982). Intellectual and adaptive performances of Asian children in adoptive American settings. *Developmental Psychology, 18,* 595–599.

Cone, C. A. (1979). Personality and subsistence: Is the child the parent of the person? *Ethnology, 18,* 291–301.

Dunnigan, T. (1982). Segmentary kinship in an urban society: The Hmong of St. Paul-Minneapolis. *Anthropological Quarterly, 55,* 126–134.

Egan, M. G. (1985). A family assessment challenge: Refugee youth and foster family adaptation. *Topics in Clinical Nursing, 7,* 64–69.

Faulkner, J., and Kich, G. K. (1983). Assessment and engagement stages in therapy with the interracial family. In J. C. Hansen and C. J. Falicov (eds.), *Cultural Perspectives in Family Therapy,* pp. 78–90. Rockville, Md.: Aspen.

Freyberg, J. (1980). Difficulties in separation-individuation as experienced by offspring of Nazi Holocaust survivors. *American Journal of Orthopsychiatry, 50,* 87–95.

Harding, R. K., and Looney, J. G. (1977). Problems of Southeast Asian children in a refugee camp. *American Journal of Psychiatry, 134,* 407–411.

Hill, D. (1975). Personality factors amongst adolescents in minority ethnic groups. *Educational Studies, 1,* 43–54.

Hoang, G. N., and Erickson, R. V. (1985). Cultural barriers to effective medical care among Indochinese patients. *Annual Review of Medicine, 36,* 229–239.

Hodson, E. M., and Springthorpe, B. J. (1976). Medical problems in refugee children evacuated from South Vietnam. *Medical Journal of Australia, 2,* 747–749.

Ionescu-Tongyonk, J. (1977). Depressions and general medicine: The depressions of childhood and adolescence. *Thai Medical Journal, 1,* 268–277.

Jalali, B., and Boyce, E. (1980). Multicultural families in treatment. *International Journal of Family Psychiatry, 1,* 475–484.

Katz, P. (1979). Salteaux-Ojibway adolescents: The adolescent process amidst a clash of cultures. *Psychiatric Journal of the University of Ottawa, 4,* 315–321.

Kelly, G. P. (1977). *From Vietnam to America.* Boulder, Colo.: Westview Press.

Kerr, H. D., and Saryan, L. A. (1986). Arsenic content of homeopathic medicines. *Clinical Toxicology, 24,* 451–459.

Kim, S. C. (1985). Family therapy for Asian Americans: A strategic-structural framework. *Psychotherapy, 22,* 342–348.

Krell, R. (1985a). Child survivors of the Holocaust: 40 years later. *Journal of the American Academy of Child Psychiatry, 24,* 378–380.

Krell, R. (1985b). Therapeutic value of documenting child survivors. *Journal of the American Academy of Child Psychiatry, 24,* 397–400.

Krell, R. (1988). Survivors of childhood experiences in Japanese concentration camps. *American Journal of Psychiatry, 145,* 383–384.

Kremer, P. G., and Sabin, C. (1985). Indochinese immigrant children: Problems in psychiatric diagnosis. *Journal of the American Academy of Child Psychiatry, 24,* 453–458.

Krupinski, J., and Burrows, G. (eds.). (1986). *The Price of Freedom: Young Indochinese in Australia.* New York: Pergamon.

Lampkin, L. C. (1971). Alienation as a coping mechanism. In E. Parrenstedt and W. Bernard (eds.), *Crisis of Family Disorganization*. New York: Behavioral Publications.

Lappin, J. (1983). On becoming a culturally conscious family therapist. In J. C. Hansen and C. J. Falicov (eds.), *Cultural Perspectives in Family Therapy*, pp. 91–107. Rockville, Md.: Aspen.

Lappin, J., and Scott, S. (1982). Intervention in a Vietnamese refugee family. In J. McGoldrick, K. Pearce, and J. Giordano (eds.), *Ethnicity and Family Therapy*, pp. 483–490. New York: Guilford Press.

Lawlor, J. (1988, January 30). Amerasians start a new life in USA. *USA Today*, p. 1.

Lee, E. (1988). Cultural factors in working with Southeast Asian refugee adolescents. *Journal of Adolescence, 11*, 167–179.

Leichty, M. M. (1963). Family attitudes and self concept in Vietnamese and U.S. children. *American Journal of Orthopsychiatry, 33*, 38–50.

Leon, G. R., Butcher, J. N., Kleinman, M., Goldberg, A., and Almagor, M. (1981). Survivors of the Holocaust and their children: Current status and adjustment. *Journal of Personality and Social Psychology, 41*, 503–516.

Levy, J. (1933). Conflicts of cultures and children's maladjustment. *Mental Hygiene, 17*, 41–50.

Lewis, P., Rack, P. H., Vaddadi, K. S., and Allen, J. J. (1980). Ethnic differences in drug response. *Postgraduate Medical Journal, Suppl. 1*, 46–49.

Livingston, R. (1987). Maternal somatization disorder and Munchausen syndrome by proxy. *Psychosomatics, 28*, 213–214.

Lopata, H. Z. (1975). A life record of an immigrant. *Society, 13*, 64–74.

Marmot, M. G., and Syme, S. L. (1976). Acculturation and coronary heart disease in Japanese-Americans. *American Journal of Epidemiology, 104*, 225–247.

McBogg, P., and Wouri, D. (1979). Outcome of adopted Vietnamese children. *Clinical Pediatrics, 18*, 179–183.

McGoldrich, M., Pearce, J., and Giordano, J. (eds.). (1982). *Ethnicity and Family Therapy*. New York: Guilford Press.

McKelvey, R.F.S. (1988). A continuum of mental health care for children and adolescents. *Hospital and Community Psychiatry, 39*, 870–873.

Moffic, H. S., Kendrick, E. A., Lomax, J. W., and Reid, K. (1987). Education in cultural psychiatry in the United States. *Transcultural Psychiatric Research Reviews, 24*, 166–187.

Morgan, M. C., Wingard, D. L., and Felice, M. E. (1984). Subcultural differences in alcohol use among youth. *Journal of Adolescent Health Care, 5*, 191–195.

Murray, D. L., Lynch, M., Doughty, A., and Cho, B. K. (1988). Results of screening adopted Korean children for HBsAg. *American Journal of Public Health, 78*, 855–856.

Naditch, M. P., and Morrissey, R. F. (1976). Role stress, personality, and psychopathology in a group of immigrant adolescents. *Journal of Abnormal Psychology, 85*, 113–118.

Nguyen, L. T., and Henkin, A. B. (1980). Reconciling differences: Indochinese refugee students in American schools. *The Clearing House, 54,* 105–108.

Okuma, T. (1981). Differential sensitivity to the effects of psychotropic drugs: Psychotics vs. normals; Asians vs. Western populations. *Folie Psychiatrica et Neurologica Japonica, 35,* 79–81.

Olness, K. (1977). The ecology of malnutrition in children. *Journal of the American Medical Womens Association, 32,* 279–284.

Patkin, S. G., Shen, Y., Pardes, H., Shu, L., Korpi, E., Wyatt, R., Phelps, B. H., and Zhou, B. (1984). Haloperidol concentrations elevated in Chinese patients. *Psychiatry Research, 12,* 167–172.

Philips, I. (1979). Childhood depression: Interpersonal interactions and depressive phenomena. *American Journal of Psychiatry, 136,* 511–513.

Rakoff, V. (1964). Children and families of concentration camp survivors. *Canada's Mental Health, 14,* 14–16.

Rathbun, C., Di Virgilio, L., and Waldfogel, S. (1958). The restitutive process in children following radical separation from family and culture. *American Journal of Orthopsychiatry, 28,* 408–415.

Rumbaut, R. D., and Rumbaut, R. G. (1976). The family in exile: Cuban expatriates in the United States. *American Journal of Psychiatry, 133,* 395–399.

Sack, W. H., Angell, R. H., Kinzie, J. D., and Rath, B. (1986). The psychiatric effects of massive trauma on Cambodian children: II. The family, the home, and the school. *Journal of the American Academy of Child Psychiatry, 25,* 377–383.

Seligman, M.E.P. (1975). *Helplessness: On Depression, Development and Death.* San Francisco: Freeman.

Shon, S. P., and Ja, D. Y. (1982). Asian families. In M. McGoldrich, J. K. Pearce, and J. Giordano (eds.), *Ethnicity and Family Therapy,* pp. 108–228. New York: Guilford.

Smyke, P. (1988). Journey into exile. *Refugees, 54,* 21–11.

Sokoloff, B., Carlin, J., and Pham, H. (1984). Five-year follow-up of Vietnamese refugee children in the United States. *Clinical Pediatrics, 23,* 565–570.

Spiegel, J. (1982). An ecological model of ethnic families. In M. McGoldrich, J. K. Pearce, and J. Giordano (eds.), *Ethnicity and Family Therapy,* pp. 31–51. New York: Guilford.

Stalcup, S. A., Oscherwitz, M., Cohen, M. S., Crast, F., Broughton, D., Stark, F., and Goldsmith, R. (1975). Planning for a pediatric disaster—experience gained from caring for 1600 Vietnamese orphans. *New England Journal of Medicine, 293,* 691–695.

Szapocznik, J., Kurtines, W. M., and Fernandez, T. (1980). Bicultural involvement and adjustment in Hispanic-American youths. *International Journal of Intercultural Relations, 4,* 355–365.

Szapocznik, J. Scopetta, M. A., Laranalde, M. A., and Kurtines, W. (1978).

Cuban value structure: Treatment implications. *Journal of Consulting and Clinical Psychology, 46,* 961–970.

Terr, L. C. (1981). Psychic trauma in children: Observations following the Chowchilla school-bus kidnapping. *American Journal of Psychiatry, 138,* 14–19.

Tobin, J. J., and Friedman, J. (1984). Intercultural and developmental stresses confronting Southeast Asian refugee adolescents. *Journal of Operational Psychiatry, 15,* 39–45.

Trossman, B. (1968). Adolescent children of concentration camp survivors. *Canadian Psychiatric Association Journal, 13,* 121–123.

Weissman, M. M., Wickramaratne, P., Warner, P., John, K., Prusoff, B. A., Merikangas, K. R., and Gammon, D. (1987). Assessing psychiatric disorders in children: Discrepancies between mothers' and childrens' reports. *Archives of General Psychiatry, 44,* 747–753.

Welner, Z. (1978). Childhood depression: An overview. *Journal of Nervous and Mental Disease, 166,* 588–593.

Westermeyer, J. (1985). Psychiatric diagnosis across cultural boundaries. *American Journal of Psychiatry, 142,* 798–805.

Westermeyer, J. (1987a). Clinical considerations in cross cultural diagnosis. *Hospital and Community Psychiatry, 38,* 160–165.

Westermeyer, J. (1987b). Cultural factors in clinical assessment. *Journal of Consulting and Clinical Psychology, 55,* 471–478.

Westermeyer, J. (1987c). Psychiatric care of refugees. In R. H. Sandler and T. C. Jones (eds.), *Medical Care of Refugees,* pp. 213–218. New York: Oxford University Press.

Westermeyer, J. (1988). DSM III psychiatric disorders among Hmong refugees in the United States: A point prevalence study. *American Journal of Psychiatry, 145,* 197–202.

Westermeyer, J. (1989). *Psychiatric Care of Migrants.* Washington, D.C.: American Psychiatric Press.

Westermeyer, J., Bouafuely, M., and Vang, T. F. (1984). Hmong refugees in Minnesota: Sex roles and mental health. *Medical Anthropology, 8,* 229–245.

Westermeyer, J., and Williams, C. (1986). Planning for mental health services for refugees. In C. Williams and J. Westermeyer (eds.), *Refugee Mental Health in Resettlement Countries,* pp. 235–245. New York: Hemisphere.

Westermeyer, R., and Westermeyer, J. (1977). Tonal language acquisition among Lao children. *Anthropological Linguistics, 19,* 260–264.

Williams, C., and Westermeyer, J. (1983). Psychiatric problems among adolescent Southeast Asian refugees: A descriptive study. *Journal of Nervous and Mental Disease, 171,* 79–85.

Williams, C. L. (1985). The Southeast Asian refugees and community mental health. *Journal of Community Psychology, 13,* 258–269.

Williamson, J. (1988). Half the world's refugees. *Refugees, 54,* 16–18.

Yang, Y. Y. (1985). Psychiatric efficacy of lithium and its effective plasma levels in Chinese bipolar patients. *Acta Psychiatrica Scandinavica, 71,* 171–175.

Young, R. C. (1983). Plasma nor$_1$-chlorpromazine concentrations: Effects of age, race, and sex. *Therapeutic Drug Monitoring, 8,* 23–26.

Ziegler, V. E., and Biggs, J. T. (1977). Tricyclic plasma levels: Effects of age, race, sex, and smoking. *Journal of the American Medical Association, 283,* 2167–2169.

8 Recovery and Rebuilding: The Challenge for Refugee Children and Service Providers

MARGARET LEIPER DE MONCHY

Since 1975, increasing numbers of refugee children and families are resettling and seeking asylum in the United States. These new members of our communities arrive with the wounds of their tragic past. They come with behaviors developed to meet the treacherous demands of survival, with broken families and communities, and with a language and culture alien to those of their new land. They also bring with them significant strengths and the hope for a bright new future, the dream that often sustained them during the hardship of their forced migration.

Unfortunately, arrival to this land of freedom does not in itself fulfill this dream. Rebuilding lives is a long, difficult process exacerbated by the new stresses and traumas of adjustment and acculturation. During resettlement, the legacy of living with terrorism and war is ever-present. Without appropriate support services and interventions, the result will be intense, violent, and costly to the survivors and to society as a whole.

This chapter addresses the challenge that today's refugee child survivors present to human service providers and systems. Emphasis is placed on the importance of integrating trauma education, cross-cultural approaches, and interagency collaboration to support the child, the child's family, and the provider throughout the delicate stages of the recovery process.

Information provided is based on the author's experience working with refugee children and their families, both in refugee camps and during resettlement. In addition, a number of individuals, including refugee paraprofessionals and professionals in the field, have contributed to the development of this chapter.

The names of individuals and certain details concerning their lives have been changed to protect their privacy.

THE REFUGEE CHILD SURVIVOR

Who is the refugee child survivor? He is the boy who studies day and night to become a doctor, the decision he made after burying his parents and siblings when he was 10 years old. She is the 13-year-old who is terrified of being alone and has no words to describe her fear. He is the 14-year-old boy who cries alone after learning from his parents in their homeland that his 9-year-old sister drowned while escaping. He is the intelligent young boy who has stolen two cars and secretly tells you where his gun is hidden. She is the teenager who never speaks above a whisper. She is the 9-year-old who misses school to take her mother to the doctor because she can speak English. They are the children who wake up, night after night, with nightmares. They are the overachievers and they are the high school dropouts. They are the children whose stories are not visible on their faces. They are the ones who learned at a young age that the world is not a safe place.

Refugee children who have survived war and violence live in a different world from other children. During the vulnerable years of childhood, they have lived in countries where terrorism and death became the norm. Most have been forced to make decisions beyond their years, when parents were no longer able to provide security and protection.

While their presence is a tribute to their resiliency and strength, they are now faced with the need to heal and to build new lives in an unfamiliar culture, with few of the natural support systems on which individuals rely following tragic life events. In addition, the values and behaviors they developed to survive in the trauma culture (of war, of exile, and of flight) often inhibit healthy development in their new world.

THE CHALLENGE OF RESETTLEMENT FOR REFUGEE SURVIVORS

All refugees and immigrants are faced with the difficult process of building new lives in an alien environment with poverty, dangerous neighborhoods, changing socioeconomic status, alienation from the dominant culture, discrimination, and struggling with intergenerational conflict due to varying rates of acculturation.

Refugees who have survived multiple losses and years of threat to their existence face unique issues in addition to those of other migrants. Some arrive with serious and chronic health needs resulting from malnutrition, lack of adequate health care, and injuries of war. In times of war and oppression, children are the most susceptible to illness and physical injury. Constant upheaval, poor sanitary conditions, and the lack of adequate nourishment leave them vulnerable to disease and malnutrition. As they secure basic needs, the psychological impact of their past trauma can begin to surface.

Additionally, values and norms of the trauma culture often continue following resettlement. Survivor communities of today struggle with issues of mistrust, corruption, and exploitation. These post-trauma and resettlement conditions recreate some experiences of the initial war trauma for children.

Loss of Parental Support and Protection

Children experience trauma in times of war and escape to a degree that depends largely on the ability of parents and other significant adults to provide security and protection. However, when terrorism and torture are used to gain absolute power over people, parents are stripped of their ability to provide protection, nourishment, and comfort. At the same time, the fear, helplessness, and stress that parents experience is passed on to the children.

During resettlement, parenting is again a difficult task. Some children watch parents become anxious, fearful, and powerless when confronted with linguistic and cultural barriers, dependency on welfare, and the exhaustion of accumulated stress. Adults are too burdened and weak to monitor children as they would under normal circumstances. Intergenerational tension due to differing rates of acculturation often results in conflict at home and further separation. All of these circumstances reinforce the belief that parents and other significant adults are not dependable and should not be trusted.

Adult Responsibility

When parents can provide limited or no protection, children are forced to fend for themselves and to make adult decisions. During war, many children become primary caretakers for younger siblings, struggling to find food and shelter in the midst of constant danger. Often, the consequences of their decisions could result in life or death.

Following resettlement, refugee children are again forced to take on adult responsibilities. Due to more rapid acculturation and command of the English language, many children and youth become the critical link between their parents and the new society. They are the ones who must communicate with landlords, doctors, school officials, and other authorities.

The majority of the recent influx of refugees come from rural, agricultural backgrounds. Some have little knowledge of the dangers of urban street life, and, consequently, do not attempt to protect their children from cars, drug pushers, and sexual offenders.

For those who are separated from their parents, the burden of parenting younger siblings continues even with the presence of other caretakers. Commitments to honor and uphold the wishes and advice of parents are strong. Conflict may develop when the mission given by parents in the homeland is unrealistic within the context of Western culture.

Vulnerability to Corruption, Promiscuity, and Abuse

Corruption, promiscuity, and abuse are inherent to circumstances of political upheaval and conflict. Children are easily coerced by those adults who promise reward and excitement. They may align themselves with the aggressors, the ones with power, the ones with food, the ones who survive.

> Here in the camp I never miss school. I like to draw and count. But I would not like to draw and count when I grow up. I'd rather be a soldier. Soldiers are not afraid of anyone. (Ek Son, 10 years old, National Federation of UNESCO Associations in Japan, 1980)

Often children are recruited as soldiers and are used to commit acts of violence against others. In the most destructive situations, they are even manipulated to inform on their own parents and friends when the consequence could be death. Children can also be physically abused and raped during escape and in refugee camps.

> Young girls who have been raped may get compassion from their relatives, support from friends, or mercy from neighbors or boat partners. But, as a girl put it, "I try to take it as an accident. But I was hurt deeply in my body and my mind. And the more people feel sorry for me, the more I feel diminished. The others are like a mirror for us." (Schroeder-Dao, 1982)

For some children and youth, the potential for continuing these patterns and being revictimized following resettlement is ever-present. With the loss of self-esteem and healthy boundaries, child survivors can be vulnerable to corruption and promiscuity on the streets in this country. Additionally, when confronted with stressful and threatening situations, some youth are forced to rely on behaviors familiar to them. Urban gang leaders take the place of soldiers. Living on the edge of life and death continues.

Addressing the needs of refugee youth and their families must include recognition of resettlement conditions that foster continuation of the trauma culture. Making the transition from beliefs, behaviors, and social systems adaptive to survival in extreme, life-threatening situations to ones that promote trust, healthy relationships, and peace is a long and delicate process. Circumstances of resettlement can impede this process. Physical health and safety are priorities. Victims are vulnerable to revictimization. Healing does not occur when demands for survival continue with great intensity.

THE CHALLENGE FOR HUMAN SERVICE PROVIDERS

Human service providers play a significant role in the refugee resettlement process. The U.S. government mandates that all legal refugees must enter this country under the auspices of a resettlement agency and must receive an initial health assessment followed by any treatment that might be indicated. Social and mental health services are often accessed later when crisis intervention becomes a necessity for some individuals and families. Recent studies indicate that prevalence rates of mental health service needs among current refugee populations are higher than those of the general population (Gong-Guy, 1987; Meinhardt et al., 1984; Westermeyer, 1986). The involvement of service providers in the post-trauma lives of child survivors can contribute to the rebuilding process or may inadvertently revictimize survivors and support the continuation of destructive patterns. The impact of the "second injury" (Symonds, 1980) to survivors of extreme trauma has been documented as profound and lasting (Danieli, 1984; Rappaport, 1968). Appropriate, sensitive, and supportive service delivery requires from providers a commitment to learn about refugees, their experiences, and their cultures, as well as willingness to be creative and flexible in the service approach.

In order to meet the challenge of providing appropriate and non-violating services, the needs of providers, when confronted with refugee clients, must also be identified and understood. For many refugee populations, there are few, if any, bilingual, bicultural professionals available. Adequate service delivery to refugee clients is therefore dependent on Western professionals. Clearly, linguistic and cultural barriers to communication are priority issues. Without the ability to communicate, collecting information and establishing a trusting relationship, essential to the helping process and effective intervention, is an impossible task. Working in teams with interpreters and paraprofessionals becomes a necessity and presents a new set of problems. Most Western professionals are not familiar with the dynamics of cross-cultural team interventions. Feelings of impotence and loss of control with clients are inevitable. Most interpreters and paraprofessionals have limited training and need support for their own acculturation and post-trauma adjustment. These needs result in additional demands on the Western professionals with respect to both time and sensitivity.

In addition, many skilled Western clinicians have had limited training in cross-cultural and post-traumatic stress issues relevant to assessment and treatment. While increasing numbers of educational programs are being developed, few service systems manage to provide these training opportunities for their staff, especially where client numbers are low. Without training and previous experience, clinicians can misinterpret symptoms, become frustrated with clients who don't trust or follow through with service plans, and may be unaware of an overwhelming number of unmet needs that impact treatment. Resulting feelings of inadequacy and helplessness for often overworked human service professionals can lead to denial of client symptoms as a means of self-protection. In some cases, countertransference issues lead to overprotective and paternalistic approaches to survivors. This can be especially damaging for refugee children whose relationship with parents is already pressured by differential rates of acculturation.

When working with refugee clients, providers also cope with the limited availability of appropriate referral resources. Effective delivery of a specialized service can be impeded and clinicians are faced with responding to needs outside the mandate of their agency's responsibility. This often results in extra hours of work for committed professionals, and sometimes in confrontations with supervisors and administrators.

Language and cultural barriers, limited training and support, lack of appropriate referral resources, and countertransference issues are problems experienced by human service providers in working with refugee clients. When not addressed, these problems can result in dangerous and inappropriate service delivery to refugee children and their families. Clinicians inadvertently create additional stress in child survivors' lives when culture and traditional beliefs are violated; when lack of involvement with parents, due to language barriers, increases alienation of children from their families; and when assessment and diagnosis are inadequate or inappropriate. To avoid inflicting additional injury to refugee youth and their families, training and careful program development is imperative.

Building Appropriate and Effective Service Delivery Systems

Planning for the development of appropriate services for refugee children involves the recognition of some fundamental principles and program components. While some of these are not unique to services for refugees, they are emphasized here because of their importance in both the acculturation process and recovery from trauma. Principles essential to effective service delivery are the following.

— Trauma experiences need to be acknowledged as they have impacted the child's development, perception of the world, and vision for the future.

— Recognizing the success of refugees as survivors, and affirming their wisdom and strengths, are essential to helping them improve their self-esteem.

— Cross-cultural living skills need to be taught in order for refugees to develop positive bicultural identities.

— Empowerment and the recovery of control over one's life need to be encouraged, especially for refugees who are reestablishing parental roles with their children.

The following are program components that incorporate these principles and contribute to helpful intervention with refugee youth and their families. They also provide opportunities for reducing some of the barriers experienced by Western professionals when working with refugees.

Use of Trained Bilingual, Bicultural Staff

Clearly, the use of trained bilingual, bicultural staff is necessary for basic communication when children have limited English language skills. Even when language proficiency increases for refugee children, their dominant language remains that of their homeland and is often the primary one spoken at home. Rapid acquisition of spoken English for refugee youth can far exceed their level of comprehension. Staff from the same ethnic background are important because of their understanding of the client's cultural base, degree of cross-cultural competence, and their ability to recognize culture-bound, nonverbal messages. This is particularly important with refugee youth who come from cultures where verbalization of emotions is not the norm.

Equally important to facilitating communication with youth is the ability of bilingual, bicultural staff to communicate with and include parents and other significant family members in the assessment and treatment processes. Too often, refugee parents are alienated from their children's lives when service systems depend solely on the use of interpreters. Both time and funds are limited. Reliance on interpreter pools prevents the development of trusting therapeutic relationships between clients and service providers and often leads to alienation, misunderstanding, and noncompliance.

Bilingual, bicultural staff become bridges between refugee communities and Western service systems. They are the conduits for increased cross-cultural understanding. Most refugees come from countries where traditional helpers are family elders, religious leaders, and indigenous helpers. While hospitals and mental health facilities might have developed following Western influence, they were limited and, for the most part, confined to urban areas. Consequently, most refugees are extremely confused by the human service system in this country. Bilingual, bicultural staff provide information to their communities about access and service procedures. They also educate Western professionals about cultural values and traditional beliefs, which assists in the prevention of unintentional violation of clients.

Cross-cultural teams are needed when bilingual, bicultural professionals are not available. Many of today's refugees come from countries where there were a limited number of professionals in the health, mental health, and social service fields. In some cases, professionals have been identified as "enemies" of a political regime and systematically eliminated. The professionals who do survive and then arrive as refugees struggle through time-consuming licensing procedures in this country. They also must cope with their own post-trauma and resettlement adjustment.

The cross-cultural team approach offers many advantages when working with refugee children who are in the process of integrating two worlds, their homeland and the adoptive country. With both a Western professional and paraprofessional from the same ethnic background, treatment can be flexible and responsive to the child's stage in the acculturation process without alienation of parents. This is especially valuable for those youth needing to reject their cultural background because of memories that produce feelings of pain and horror or guilt and shame. Teams can be a visible symbol of integration, with respect for both cultures. In addition, they provide support and training to refugee paraprofessional staff whose expertise has come from experience rather than formal education in Western disciplines.

Knowledge of Refugee Trauma Experiences and Post-trauma Syndromes

Providing services that effectively meet the needs of refugee children who have been victimized by war and traumatized by escape and relocation requires the recognition and understanding of the effects of these experiences on their psychological, emotional, and physical lives.

Knowledge of post-trauma symptoms and their impact on families and communities is also essential for successful understanding and validation of a child's natural support systems.

There is a growing body of research on the psychological impact of both traumatic life events and the refugee experience. Studies on the consequences of trauma experienced during childhood indicate that the *Diagnostic and Statistical Manual of Mental Disorders*, 3rd ed. revised (*DSM-IIIR*) criteria for post-traumatic stress disorder recognized in adults can also be directly applied to children (Eth and Pynoos, 1985). Recent research by Eth and Pynoos (1985) indicates that post-trauma recovery for the child results in important developmental influences on behavior, cognition, and emotion. They conclude that, "Recognition of . . . phase salient differences is critical for the understanding of traumatic effects on personality and the implementation of developmentally sound treatment strategies." Research specific to the refugee child's experience identifies the additional impact of pervasive, multiple traumas and forced migration on refugee children. An annotated bibliography on refugee mental health provides a comprehensive listing of literature relevant to this subject through 1986 (Williams, 1987).

Training in post-traumatic stress theory and the refugee experience provides an opportunity for Western clinicians to develop awareness of their own reactions and countertransference issues. This is critical to working with survivors. Much of the violation identified as the "second injury" (Symonds, 1980) or the "trauma after trauma" (Rappaport, 1968) occurs when well-intentioned professionals unconsciously deny or obsess over a client's trauma experience. This also happens when clinicians become paternalistic and overprotective and fail to acknowledge the survivor's dignity and strengths.

Linkage with Refugee Communities

Essential to the responsiveness and credibility of any program providing services to refugees is an established linkage with community leaders and representatives. Because these communities are often fragmented and have a number of factions, each with its own power base and ideology, a single leader may not represent the entire community. Therefore, it is important for service providers to become aware of the unique identities and dynamics within the communities they are serving.

There are several advantages in this linkage to ensuring effective delivery of services to refugee children. First, it provides an informal sanction of the service because the community has an opportunity to understand the service as one that may be beneficial. This is especially important because most refugees are unfamiliar with Western concepts of human service delivery. This lack of understanding combined with the apprehension and mistrust of authorities fostered by the refugee experience can lead to suspicion of human service workers. Social workers responsible for child protective services may be viewed as the enemy because they sometimes take children away. Unfamiliar hospital procedures can be perceived as harmful, and mental health professionals may talk about painful experiences which, according to tradition, should be left to rest and not discussed. Second, through established linkages, service providers have the opportunity to be aware of significant events that occur in the larger refugee community and potentially impact the child.

Finally, this linkage offers opportunities to enhance redevelopment of the natural support systems of children. Through communication and a greater understanding of the community, service providers convey, to both parents and children, respect for their cultural identity and traditions.

Integration of Traditional Methods of Healing

The issue of traditional healing must be addressed when considering the development of appropriate and culturally sensitive services to meet the needs of the recent influx of refugees. This is particularly important for survivors whose need for familiar, natural support systems is so essential to rebuilding and recovery following extreme loss. The majority of today's refugees come from countries where traditional concepts of illness and healing are vastly different than those of this country. Illness, especially mental illness, as well as some social problems are believed to be a result of spiritual wrongdoings in this life or a previous life. Thus healing rituals incorporate methods of asking for forgiveness from ancestors and higher spirits and acknowledging their power. For Southeast Asians, physical illness is directly related to an imbalance both in one's body and in the harmony of body, mind, and spirit. Healing involves opening "blockages" to allow the blood and air to flow freely and return heat energy evenly throughout the body. In addition, herbal medicine is used to relieve symptoms and recover a healthy state. Refugees in this country continue to use traditional methods of healing in their homes, religious institutions, and in the homes of traditional healers.

Integration of traditional methods of healing into health and human service delivery to refugees, when appropriate, can enhance the effectiveness of the treatment. Recognition of traditional healing and religious practices can also prevent some refugees from resisting Western treatment when it may be necessary. The following case illustrates this point:

Case 1: A 17-year-old Cambodian boy was hospitalized one week after his arrival in the United States as an unaccompanied minor. He was diagnosed as having severe sclerosis of the liver as a result of untreated hepatitis B and immediately placed in isolation with the requirement that all staff and visitors must wear gowns, gloves, and masks when entering his room. There were no bilingual, bicultural staff available at the hospital and communication was only possible during visits from a social worker and a Cambodian paraprofessional. On the third day following admission, the patient suddenly became unmanageable. He was found cowering under his bed, pulling his intravenous line out of his arm and wrapping the tubing around his neck as if to strangle himself. Following extensive psychological testing which further agitated the young man and produced no indication of the cause of his behavior, the social worker was permitted to talk with him. She discovered that he was "seeing" his mother, grandmother, and four friends, all of whom had died during the Pol Pot regime, surround his bed and call him to join them. He also saw many white ghosts in the room. This was terrifying to him and an indication that he would die soon. With the help of the Cambodian paraprofessional, it was determined that he believed strongly in the power of ancestors and in the protection offered by blessings from the monks. Arrangements were made for a Cambodian monk to come to the hospital room and perform a ceremony of protection around the patient. A knotted string, blessed by holy water, was tied around his waist and an altar was set up next to his bed. Following this ritual, the young man was compliant with treatment and responsive to medication.

Generalizations about refugee children and adolescents' beliefs in traditional healing are difficult to make. Young children adopt the beliefs of parents and other significant adults who tend to cling to the old traditions. Later, after entry into the Western educational system and during the process of developing their own cross-cultural identities, refugee youth may fluctuate between both traditions. Many factors impact the beliefs of bicultural children and youth, including memories from childhood and the effectiveness of past treatments, relationships with parents, attitudes toward the culture as a whole, and level of security. In some instances, traditional beliefs have been adopted even when they are unfamiliar to the young person. This happens most often with children who have lost or been separated from parents at a young age.

An understanding of traditional rituals, methods of healing, and religious beliefs can be important to appropriate diagnosis. Some methods of healing produce bruises that have been misinterpreted as signs of child abuse. In other cases, refugee youth in mental health facilities have been seen as exhibiting self-destructive behavior because they shaved their heads and eyebrows to offer a sacrifice to ancestors whom they may have wronged.

Bilingual, bicultural staff are essential to ascertaining the client's particular belief system. They also provide education regarding the appropriate use of traditional healing to Western staff and, most importantly, provide access to traditional healers when necessary.

INTEGRATION OF SPECIALIZED SERVICES INTO A COMPREHENSIVE SERVICE SYSTEM

One of the most significant impediments to providing effective services to refugees is the highly specialized and bureaucratized nature of our service delivery system. For refugees with multiple needs, the complexity and fragmentation of our system can be overwhelming. Service providers working with refugees encounter these complexities as well. Limited resources and lack of appropriate services impact the providers' capacity to assist their clients to meet basic life needs or other specialized needs. This results in the inevitable feeling, on the part of providers, that they are helpless and ineffective in sufficiently meeting the needs of their clients.

For refugees, the structure of our service system is often perceived as not helpful. They are used to traditional systems where interventions were more holistic and, therefore, provided more immediate results. The protocols established as normal procedures in this country for determining individual needs are often cumbersome and not necessarily designed to respond immediately to the immediate problem.

To reduce these inherent barriers in a fragmented system, specialized services to refugees must be provided within the context of the comprehensive service system. Collaborative planning will ensure that linkages are established that facilitate efficient access to all needed services. These collaborative efforts also foster important relationships among service providers and, therefore, facilitate referral processes and diminish feelings of isolation.

SERVICE MODELS

Providing services that effectively address the needs of refugee child survivors presents unique challenges to the service delivery system. It is important that a balance between mainstream and specialized services be achieved. While the availability of interpreters is fundamental to improving access to existing services for refugee clients, this service alone is not sufficient to provide quality care.

Developing a comprehensive system of services to meet the special-

ized needs of refugee clients requires collaborative efforts between public agencies and the private sector. Services to refugee children and
youth cannot be provided in isolation from their parents and families.
Programs must be supported, not only with fiscal and staff resources,
but also through federal and state policies that reflect an understanding
of the unique needs of these communities and a solid commitment to
providing culturally and linguistically appropriate services.

It is important to acknowledge that services to refugee clients are
cost-intensive. Refugees comprise a relatively small percentage of a total
client population, but have specialized service needs. Cross-cultural
teams are essential to providing quality intervention and care for some
refugee groups, but are an additional cost. Specialized training must
also be available for staff and provider agencies serving refugee communities. Therefore, cost-sharing among public and private agencies is
extremely advantageous in the development of a comprehensive service
delivery system.

Models in Massachusetts

In response to the influx of refugees, primarily from Southeast Asia, the
Commonwealth of Massachusetts has developed some innovative specialized services. Two, in particular, have incorporated many of the components previously identified that contribute to effective delivery of
services to refugee child survivors and their families.

The following program models represent two different approaches to
the delivery of culturally and linguistically appropriate, comprehensive
child welfare, health, and mental health services. One serves a wide
geographic area and works collaboratively with local service agencies
providing an opportunity to respond to the mobility of the client population. The other is a community-based clinic that provides an array of
services in the client's own neighborhood.

Metropolitan Indochinese Children and Adolescent Services (MICAS). MICAS
is a program that provides child welfare and mental health services to
Cambodian, Laotian, and Vietnamese children and adolescents. Its services range from school- and home-based adjustment counseling to intensive hospital diversion and inpatient psychiatric support. With this
broad range of service components, staff are able to follow a client and
the client's family through the complexities of the bureaucratic system
without disrupting often delicate therapeutic relationships.

MICAS services are provided across a wide geographic region. While
the central office is located in Chelsea, a community near Boston that
is densely populated by Southeast Asian refugees, satellite sites are

located in various schools with significant Southeast Asian student populations. MICAS is a program of the South Cove Community Health Center, which serves primarily the Chinese population of greater Boston. This base in an established and reputable ethnic community agency provides resources and facilitates the procedure of contracting for funds. The program operates with funds from the State Departments of Education, Social Services, and Mental Health; from two United Ways of Massachusetts; from private foundations; and from the cities of Boston and Chelsea. Being funded to provide comprehensive services in schools, homes, and mental health facilities enables MICAS to follow and respond to the various needs of refugee child survivors through the different stages of the recovery and adjustment process. This continuity in provision of services allows refugee children to develop trust in their helpers. The cross-agency funding model provides a cost-effective method for state agencies to address the specialized service needs of a relatively small client population.

The "cross-cultural team" approach is central to the MICAS service delivery model. Each client and his or her family is assigned a Western clinician and a bilingual, bicultural paraprofessional of the same ethnic background as the client. Team members work together and independently, based on the nature of the intervention and the training level of the paraprofessional. For example, an intervention with a suicidal adolescent would always require team intervention, while counseling for intergenerational conflict might involve sessions where the paraprofessional meets independently with the child and family. In all cases, team members consult with each other on a regular basis. A full-time clinical coordinator and a full-time clinical supervisor manage, supervise, train, and support direct service staff.

Staff recruitment, development, and retention are priority concerns of MICAS. Linkages with other refugee providers, state agencies, educational institutions, and refugee community leaders are maintained to advocate for and contribute to the development of paraprofessional and cross-cultural training programs. In addition, three part-time consultants provide case consultation and training to the program staff. These include a clinical psychologist, a licensed independent clinical social worker (LICSW) with expertise in child welfare and refugee resettlement, and an LICSW experienced in teaching English as a second language with a clinical focus. Recently, MICAS has developed advancement levels for paraprofessional case workers. These standardized levels allow for goal setting with paraprofessional staff and provide incentives for skills development. Advancement directly affects defined salary increases and work assignments. Improved skills development of bilingual, bicultural staff also has program cost implications as the number of independent staff hours, versus team hours, are increased.

Linkage with the comprehensive service system and with refugee community organizations is primarily established (and maintained) through involvement in state- and city-level planning and advocacy for refugee issues. The MICAS program director devotes a considerable amount of time to this effort. Collaboration and cooperation with public service agencies contributes to both funding for MICAS services and the development of culturally appropriate and accessible referral resources for clients. Participation in ethnic community events and celebrations builds trust, mutual understanding, and cooperation between Western program staff and the communities of new Americans they serve.

Lynn Community Health Center. Lynn Community Health Center is a community-based, nonprofit corporation whose mission is to provide for the health and well-being of the residents of the greater Lynn area and surrounding communities. Since its establishment in 1973, the center has maintained a special commitment to provide high-quality care at appropriate cost to minority and low-income populations, including local cultural and linguistic minorities. In recent years, they have expanded their bilingual, bicultural staff to respond to the needs of a growing Cambodian community in the area.

The Health Center is based on the philosophy that "a healthy individual is the result of a healthy family and a healthy environment." A wide range of services are provided at multiple sites easily accessible by public transportation. These services include child/adolescent and adult medical facilities; family planning; obstetrics and gynecology; child/adolescent and adult mental health; social services; a Women, Infants, and Children (WIC) program, targeted to mother and child groups at risk for nutritional deficiencies; preventive health education; dental and vision care referral; and an on-site laboratory. With this wide range of services available at one location, the comprehensive needs of individuals and families are addressed in a holistic and accessible manner. Common cultural barriers related to confusion with a highly specialized system are reduced and clients are able to develop familiarity with and trust in providers.

The clinical staff reflect the multicultural client population served. At present, 18.5 percent of the health, mental health, and WIC program staff are bilingual, bicultural professionals and paraprofessionals. All services to bicultural clients are provided by professionals of the same ethnic background or by cross-cultural teams with an "ethnically same" paraprofessional. Flexibility in direct service hours has been established with the realization that intake information and client histories might take longer for clients not familiar with the Western service delivery system or fearful of the procedures.

Recognition that cultural issues are extremely relevant to health and mental health care has led to the development of other program components. A health educator has been hired to ensure that education and training on cross-cultural issues is emphasized for clinic staff. This component supports all staff by increasing awareness and facilitating sometimes difficult cross-cultural team work relationships. In addition, clinical teams work in the community to effect linkages with leaders of the minority groups, church leaders, school personnel, and representatives of minority serving agencies. This process also increases awareness and cross-cultural understanding, as well as building bridges critical to the effective delivery of services.

For refugee children specifically, this service model offers many healthy supports and reduces the chance of cultural and family violation. As with MICAS, the availability of bilingual, bicultural staff and cross-cultural teams provides appropriate communication for information gathering and assessment, flexibility to respond to varying levels of acculturation, comfort for children and youth less familiar with the Western culture, and most important, the link to parents and community. Perhaps the most significant advantage of the community-based model is the opportunity to track children and identify needs that might be overlooked by parents overly stressed by post-trauma adjustment and resettlement. Following initial health assessments, referral for additional services is less demanding for parents when provided in the same location and with the assistance of the same bilingual, bicultural staff previously encountered. Events occurring in the family or community that may affect the health and mental health of young clients are often known to the clinic staff. The community health center is the Western health and human services delivery model that most resembles that of traditional systems of helpers in the homelands of today's refugees.

CONCLUSION

Addressing the specialized needs of refugee children and youth presents a challenge to health and human service providers and systems. Sensitivity to early experiences of extreme trauma and understanding of cultural orientations are critical to adequate and effective helping, healing, and support. For refugee child survivors, recovery and rebuilding involves the integration of three cultures: the traditional culture, the trauma culture, and the American culture. Human service providers and programs must have the capability to support the values of all three cultures with the flexibility necessary to respond to the changing needs of children, youth, and their families.

It is important to remember that, above all, refugee children and their families are survivors. They possess tremendous strength to recover and rebuild their lives and their communities. They need information, encouragement, and support. While all child survivors must learn to live with the consequences of their traumatic past, only some need acute intervention in this process.

Survivors also have a message to give to the world. Moffat and Moffat, in *Families after Trauma* (1984), captured the value of the message refugee child survivors bring to us:

> Survivors are the bridge between the past and the future. Their experiences have given them a view of life to be shared in order to spur personal and social change. [They] are the voices that challenge complacency and the denial of reality as they know it. (p. 201)

Refugee children and other survivors are our teachers. We must listen and learn from them with respect, dignity, and compassion.

> I have come to realize that I am alive again. I am not just alive because bullets failed to reach my brain. I am not just alive because a stick missed my skull. I am alive really only because finally and painfully after these years, I know that I can love again. I can feel the suffering of others, not just my own. (Arn Chorn, Crisp, 1988)

REFERENCES

American Psychiatric Association (1987). *Diagnostic and Statistical Manual of Mental Disorders*, 3rd ed. rev. Washington, D.C.: Author.

Crisp, J. (1988). Refugee children: Policy and practice. *Refugees, 54* (June), p. 20.

Danieli, Y. (1984). Psychotherapists' participation in the conspiracy of silence about the Holocaust. *Psychoanalytic Psychology, 1*(1), 23–42.

Eth, S., and Pynoos, R. S. (1985). Developmental perspective on psychic trauma in childhood. In C. R. Figley (ed.), *Trauma and Its Wake*. New York: Brunner/Mazel.

Gong-Guy, E. (1987). *California Southeast Asian Mental Health Needs Assessment*. California State Department of Mental Health Pub. No. 85-76282A-2.

Meinhardt, K., Tom, S., Tse, P., and Yu, C. Y. (1984). Santa Clara County

Health Department Asian Health Assessment Project. Unpublished manuscript.

Moffat, L. F., and Moffat, J. G., II (1984). *Families after Trauma: An Education and Human Resource.* White Bear Lake, MN: Minnesota State Board of Vocational Technical Education.

National Federation of UNESCO Associations in Japan. (1980). *Kampuchean Chronicles.* Bangkok: Koksai Printing.

Rappaport, E. A. (1968). Beyond traumatic neurosis: A psychoanalytic study of late reactions to the concentration camp trauma. *International Journal of Psycho-Analysis, 49,* 719–731.

Schroeder-Dao, T. K. (1982). Study of rape victims among the refugees on Pulau Bidong Island: An experience in counseling women refugee "boat people." Geneva. Unpublished report.

Symonds, M. (1980). The "second injury" to victims. *Evaluation and Change 1* (Special Issue), 36–38.

Westermeyer, J. (1986). Indochinese refugees in community and clinic: A report from Asia and the United States. In C. L. Williams and J. Westermeyer (eds.), *Refugee Mental Health in Resettlement Countries,* pp. 113–130.

Williams, C. L. (1987). *An Annotated Bibliography on Refugee Mental Health.* U.S. Department of Health and Human Services publication ADM 87-1517. Washington, D.C.: National Institute of Mental Health.

9 School and the Passage of Refugee Youth from Adolescence to Adulthood

TIMOTHY READY, Ph.D.

Schools can play a crucial role in the adaptation of immigrant and refugee youths who have serious and pressing problems when they settle into their new communities. In addition to their core task of education, schools can provide career training and job placement services, language instruction, and personal and academic counseling. For those needs that the schools may not be able to address directly, such as housing, legal, health, and mental health services, educators can make referrals to other organizations. Educational institutions that take into account the needs and unique sensibilities of newly arrived immigrant and refugee youths have the potential not only to facilitate the personal adaptation of individual students, but also to play a key role in the harmonious integration of immigrant communities into the economic and social systems of the host society. The Multicultural Career Intern program[1] (MCIP) of Washington, D.C., was established specifically to accomplish these ambitious objectives: to address the needs of Washington's rapidly growing population of immigrant and refugee adolescents.

In the 1960s and 1970s a small Latino community, numerically dominated by Central Americans, was beginning to establish itself in Washington. This early migration to the city was led primarily by women (Cohen 1979, 1980), many of whom found employment as domestic workers and commercial housekeepers. As the violence in Central America worsened in the late 1970s and early 1980s, many young people chose Washington as a place of refuge because of the presence of relatives already in the city and the strong economy of the region. Some left their countries to avoid being caught up in the military conflicts that were occurring. Others were unable to continue their education because

---

[1] In 1987 the name was changed to Bell Multicultural High School. The school is now part of the District of Columbia Public School System.

their schools had been bombed or teachers assassinated. Still others left because of the increasingly desperate economic conditions.

Unlike the better-known international residents of Washington who had come to work in the embassies or international organizations such as the World Bank, most of the newcomers in the early 1980s were motivated by acute "push factors" such as the threat of war-related violence and associated economic problems (Inda, 1981). Although most refugees who arrived in Washington came from Central America, especially El Salvador, many also came from Vietnam, Cambodia, Afghanistan, and Ethiopia. This chapter describes how MCIP, the school that many of these youths attended in the early 1980s, attempted to meet the needs of refugee and immigrant adolescents. After briefly describing the school and its programs as they existed in the early 1980s, the effectiveness of MCIP will be discussed in terms of the education and employment of its former Spanish-speaking students in 1988, several years after they left the school.

MCIP: A SCHOOL FOR AT-RISK ADOLESCENTS

When MCIP began operations in 1980, a large number of Hispanic youths were coming of age in Washington for the first time in the history of the city. Hispanic Washingtonians suffered from a high rate of poverty—35 percent—roughly twice the rate for black residents, who composed 70 percent of the city's population (Singh, McGivern, and D'Emilio, 1981). Given the fact that most Washington Hispanics were newcomers, it is perhaps not surprising that so many were living in poverty. However, Hispanic leaders and others were concerned that, unless dramatic action were taken, many of the young newcomers, Hispanic and non-Hispanic, would become trapped in the poverty in which most lived when they first arrived.

Under the auspices of a Hispanic organization called SEP (translated as Jobs for Progress), these Hispanic leaders applied for and received the initial funding for MCIP from the U.S. Department of Labor. The funding came from a demonstration grant whose purpose was to replicate the success of the Career Intern Program (CIP) model, first developed in Philadelphia by the Reverend Leon Sullivan and Opportunities Industrialization Centers of America (OICA). The original CIP served educationally at-risk black American students. The primary objective of the CIP model is to prevent high school students from dropping out by demonstrating the value of schooling through career-oriented curricula, intensive counseling, and internships (Opportunities Industrialization Centers of America, 1982). The Department of Labor funded five CIP programs around the country for a period of 3 years.

MCIP was the first application of the CIP model in a multicultural setting comprised primarily of Spanish-speaking immigrants and refugees.

Having left behind the severe problems they had faced in their native countries, the youths in this study were immediately confronted with a new set of problems on their arrival in Washington, D.C. Among the more serious were the following:

— Although many sought refuge in Washington, D.C., from the war-related problems of their native countries, few were recognized by the U.S. government as refugees. Many were concerned about being caught by immigration authorities and feared what awaited them if they had to return to their native countries. Because many were undocumented aliens, they sometimes worked under blatantly exploitative conditions.

— Often at a very young age, these youths were responsible for earning enough money to support themselves while simultaneously attending high school. Although the value of education was widely recognized, attending school was sometimes considered a luxury because of the pressing need to work.

— Some youths had no close family members in the Washington area to rely on for either material or emotional support.

— Many had to adjust to living in families that had been "reconstructed," their families having been split apart during the migration process. This sometimes led to domestic discord.

— Nearly all young people had to adjust to an unfamiliar language and culture.

— Many feared for the safety of family and friends who remained in the home country.

The three main components of MCIP's program were specifically designed to assist immigrant and refugee youths to make the transition to life in the United States. The components are:

1. Multiculturalism as a central theme of the curriculum and extra-curricular activities

2. Counseling

3. Career development

Multiculturalism

MCIP functioned as an explicitly multicultural school. Through its curriculum and extracurricular activities, the school reinforced to its students the value of their native language and culture. MCIP coordinated extracurricular programs featuring the music, dance, and art of the countries represented at the school. It also sponsored a championship soccer team. For many refugee boys, playing soccer provided a unique opportunity to demonstrate some of the skills that they had been developing since childhood to others in their new society.

The school's language policy was eclectic and pragmatic. Incoming students first enrolled in a series of courses that provided instruction in English as a Second Language. Although students could not earn high school credits for their work in these courses, MCIP allowed those with limited proficiency in English to simultaneously take other courses that would allow them to make progress toward their high school diploma. This was especially important for the many youths who already were older than most U.S. high school students; it was unlikely that they could afford to remain in school if they did not graduate before age 20. Since most teachers were bilingual, instructors taught courses such as art, physical education, and mathematics in both English and Spanish. Other courses, such as Spanish grammar and Latin American history, were taught entirely in Spanish. As their English proficiency increased, students began taking other courses such as American history, literature, and English composition. The rate at which students could progress through the curriculum also was accelerated by the fact that MCIP was open year-round.

The MCIP curriculum was designed to keep immigrant and refugee youths in school by gradually increasing their exposure to the new language and culture. Students were taught that taking pride in their cultural heritage was not inconsistent with successful participation in the economic, social, and political institutions of their new country. Even though most of the students were economically poor, the message was communicated that "making it" in Washington did not require the denial of who they were or where they came from.

Counseling

Although there were only 250 students enrolled at MCIP when participants in this study were present in 1982, the school employed five counselors—far more than most high schools of comparable size. Because of the accessibility of counselors, students were able to receive the individualized attention that they very much needed. Students received academic, career, and often personal counseling from the same individual, whom they got to know very well. Counselors frequently became involved in the many practical problems of their advisees, such as needs for housing or health care. They assisted students and their families by making referrals to other agencies that provided such services. Counselors met formally with students at least once a month to review their progress. Many met with students informally much more often, as the counseling room was a popular gathering place after school and during breaks between classes. Like the teachers, most MCIP counselors were bilingual, and some came from the same countries as the students. Many of the students developed such close ties with their counselors and some of their teachers that they often related to them as if they were surrogate parents. When interviewed in 1988, many study participants related stories about how their counselors and teachers had played an important role in assisting them in overcoming a variety of difficulties. This personal involvement was especially important for those students who came to Washington alone, or who had poor relationships with parents or guardians. The fact that refugee youths attending MCIP could receive a wide variety of services in one location from people whom they knew and trusted proved to be an effective way to provide needed services to the youths and their families.

Career Development

Although MCIP and other CIPs emphasized the relevance of education for future work, the CIP model differed in its objectives from the typical vocational high school. Each student designed a career development plan in conjunction with his or her counselor. This plan guided students in their choices of classes and career internships. The career development plan included a description of a career goal and a list of the courses and types of internships that would help the student to achieve the goal. Most students expressed interest in professional employment, or jobs that required postsecondary education.

Unlike vocational schools, MCIP did not directly provide students with vocational instruction that would prepare them to enter specific careers, except for classes in typing and word processing. All students were required to take a course called the Career Counseling Seminar. In it, students learned about the kinds of work done in different careers, how to fill out job applications, and the expectations of employers. All students also participated in two brief hands-on experiences in which they "shadowed" persons working in careers of interest. For example, a student with an interest in business might spend one week observing and assisting the manager of a restaurant, and a second week in the administrative offices of a major corporation. A student interested in health care might spend one week at a medical clinic and a second week in a dental office. After completing each hands-on experience, students were required to write a summary of what they had learned, including a description of the work that was observed and the types of skills necessary to do that work.

Many MCIP students also participated in paid internships. These internships were supported by the Washington Private Industry Council, by individual employers, and by funds from federal and local job training programs. These paid internships were available only to legal residents. MCIP also coordinated internships for young people who already had graduated or who had dropped out of school. The following programs, funded through the federal Job Training and Partnership Act (JTPA), were administered by MCIP:

— Bilingual and Vocational Training Program (BVT)

— Training and Employment Program (TREP)

— On the Job Training Program (OJT)

— Stay in School Program

— Out of School Program

— Work Experience Program (WEX)

— Summer Youth Employment Program (SYEP)

MCIP referred some students to public vocational schools to pursue part-time studies in office management, auto mechanics, or other fields.

Data Collection

Initial contact with the school and its students was made in 1982. At that time, nearly all MCIP students participated in a study of the adaptation of immigrants and refugee youths. Two hundred and fifty youths from 26 different countries were enrolled at MCIP at that time. Two-thirds were from Latin America, and nearly one-half were from a single country—El Salvador. Most had been in Washington only a short time, having arrived with little or no knowledge of English, and no more understanding of life in the United States than could be learned from the movies and occasional contact with friends or family members who had been there.

Participants in the 1982 study completed questionnaires asking about the circumstances of their migration, the educational and employment status of their parents in their countries of origin and in Washington, their ability to communicate in English, psychosocial adjustment to their new environment, and their hopes for the future. In addition, the author conducted interviews and engaged in participant observation at the school in 1982 and 1983. Interviews and observations were focused on the social and cultural aspects of the transitions, or passages, that the students were going through, and the role of the school in this process.

In 1988, an attempt was made to locate the 181 Spanish-speaking participants from the 1982 study to learn how these former MCIP students had done in their education and employment. At least 145 (80 percent) were still living in metropolitan Washington, D.C., in 1988. Interviews were conducted with 112 (77 percent) of the Washington area residents. The interviews elicited detailed information on the educational and employment histories of informants since leaving MCIP. In addition to these in-depth interviews, basic information on the employment and educational status of 33 other Hispanic members of the original study population were obtained. Altogether, employment data were gathered through interviews and other sources for 76 men and 70 women, or 146 (81 percent) of the original 181 Hispanic participants from the 1982 study. Data on postsecondary education were gathered for 73 men and 73 women.

Reliable information regarding graduation from high school, including the status of persons who attended other high schools after MCIP and those who received a General Equivalence Degree (GED), was obtained for 99 percent of persons still residing in the Washington area and 91 percent of the original 181 participants in the 1982 study. Despite the innovative design of MCIP, only 61 percent had graduated from high school or received a GED by 1988. Of these, 87 percent graduated from MCIP, 8 percent from another high school, and 5 percent had earned a GED. The likelihood of completing high school was statistically unrelated to gender, socioeconomic status, the absence of either or both parents from the household, or any other social characteristics of the student about which information was recorded.

The 41 interviewees who did not graduate from high school were asked why they had dropped out. Many cited more than one reason for leaving school. The most commonly cited explanations were

— Need to work and economic necessity (34 percent)

— Loss of interest and peer pressure (27 percent)

— Pregnancy, marriage, or both (24 percent)

— Repeated academic failure (10 percent)

Other factors not mentioned by dropouts during the interviews, but that certainly contributed to school withdrawal were

— Low level of basic academic skills. Most study participants had very low standardized test scores in mathematical and verbal skills when they entered MCIP, even when tested in Spanish.

— Age. Many students, already in their late teens and early twenties, were still in high school. Some had been out of school for several years before enrolling in MCIP because of war-related disruptions.

— Language. Some youths had difficulty learning English.

— Family problems. Domestic conflict sometimes distracted students from their work.

Most interviewees—even those who did not graduate—said they believed that MCIP had been a good school for them. When interviewed in 1988, 80 percent of 106 study participants expressing an opinion about their experiences at the school were happy with how the school had served them, 8 percent had a "mixed" opinion, and 12 percent were unhappy with the school. The supportive environment of the school was most commonly cited (by 34 persons) as most beneficial. MCIP's career development program was the next most frequently cited feature (26 persons). English language learning was mentioned frequently as a positive feature (21 individuals).

Of those who were displeased with their experiences at the school, language learning was the most often cited complaint. Although classes were in English, the fact that most of the staff was bilingual and most of the students spoke Spanish was cited by eight people as having delayed their learning of English or impeded their mastery of academic subjects. The culturally and linguistically congruous (Spanish-dominant) atmosphere of the school, which may have eased the transition of many refugee youths to their new environment, was criticized by others as being "too comfortable." The role that MCIP has played in the lives of some of its Hispanic students is illustrated by the cases of Tomás, Rosalba, and Felipe.

Tomás is one of the students who was somewhat critical of MCIP. He is a graduate who in 1988 worked delivering airline tickets for a travel agency. Regarding the advantages and disadvantages of the predominantly Hispanic environment of MCIP, Tomás stated

MCIP was OK, but I think that it was a disadvantage for me with the language. I have been here eight years and I still have a strong accent. I know lots of people who came after I did who have better English. I would have learned more at another type of school. All the people around there speaking Spanish put me back. But I think that, at that time, it gave me good self-esteem. I know some kids who went to regular schools and flunked out because they couldn't talk to their friends. Regular schools can be very challenging; but if you can face it, you learn more.

Rosalba, like Tomás, also came from a rural village in El Salvador. While a student at MCIP, she lived in a small apartment with her parents and five brothers and sisters. In 1988, Rosalba described herself as having been very shy in high school and unwilling to risk speaking English. She explained how she had twice flunked the Career Counseling Seminar, the course that she thought was the most valuable to her, because she could not speak English in class. Rosalba graduated from MCIP in 1983, although she came very close to dropping out. At the age of 18, while still a student, she became pregnant and married the father, whom she had known in elementary school in El Salvador. After she married, her husband and others in her family pressured her to quit school. Ms. Davis, a counselor at MCIP, was the only person Rosalba felt she could talk to about her problems. A few months after graduating, Rosalba had her baby.

By the time her baby was born it was already becoming clear that her marriage was not working out. She became very depressed. Although ambitious and strong-willed, Rosalba feared that her hopes of going to college and becoming a lawyer would never be realized. She separated from her husband and went to work for the next three years cleaning commercial buildings. In 1987 Rosalba returned to MCIP for the first time since graduating to talk with Ms. Davis, her former counselor. Ms. Davis told her that the school ran a program called WEX. Although she would be paid only $3.50 an hour, $1.50 less than she was making as a hotel housekeeper, she would receive six months of on-the-job training and would then have a good chance of getting a better job. While still in high school, Rosalba had received some training in office management. Because of her family commitments, however, she had never worked in this field. After six months in the WEX program, Rosalba was hired as a secretary by the city government.

In 1988, Rosalba was promoted to a more responsible position and given a raise from $13,500 to $18,500 a year. Besides this job, Rosalba also worked two other part-time jobs for a total of 75 hours a week. Her mother helped her with the care of her daughter. Although she was working more hours than she would have liked, Rosalba was proud of what she had accomplished. She still hoped to become a lawyer and was optimistic that one day she would be able to do it.

Another graduate, Felipe, came to Washington, D.C., in 1981. Prior to that he had lived with his mother, a public health nurse in rural El Salvador. Because of the war, Felipe's mother sent him to join his cousins who were already living in Washington. After arriving, Felipe experienced serious difficulties adjusting to life in the city. Shortly after he arrived, a bus on which his mother was riding in El Salvador was sprayed with machine gun fire. Several passengers died; his mother was one of the few who were injured. A few months later, his mother was kidnapped by fighters who needed her nursing services. It was only several weeks later that Felipe learned that his mother had been released unharmed.

Meanwhile, in Washington, Felipe had little contact with his cousins. He shared an apartment with some newfound friends and worked full-time in a restaurant as a busboy, earning less than the minimum wage. He supported himself by working full-time while attending MCIP. Not surprisingly, Felipe was having difficulties adjusting to his new environment and sought help from one of the counselors at the school. Felipe made these comments in 1988 about how MCIP helped him to overcome his difficulties in adjusting.

Ana is now my friend but she used to be my counselor [at MCIP]. . . . She helped me a lot when I really got screwed up. I used to get on a bus and wonder what the people were thinking about me. Like, "That is just an Indian—a stupid guy." . . . I was getting sick because of the things I was seeing. . . . I was seeing everything from a racial point of view, but not from other points of view. I used to talk to Ana about it and she would understand.

I realized that I'm not the only one here in this situation. There are so many other people who must feel like me, Latinos and others. Now I don't think about it at all. I still notice [racial affronts] but I just don't think about it.

Since graduating, Felipe has been working, sometimes as a volunteer and sometimes for pay, in a variety of social service programs coordinated by Hispanic agencies in Washington. He would like to continue working within his community and eventually to get involved in politics. In 1988, Felipe continued to support himself by working as a busboy while taking classes at a local college to enter the same profession as his mother: nursing.

Most study participants perceived MCIP as an accessible, supportive place, and many former students like Rosalba and Felipe continued to identify strongly with the school years after leaving. MCIP's nurturing climate, job training program, and other services helped create a sense of community. Most youths who were associated with the school came to identify with the functional and wholesome values that the school promoted and avoided most dysfunctional attractions tempting urban youth. Although by 1988 most had not progressed far in their formal education, they were very industrious and used to good advantage the career training they received in high school.

More than half of the 112 interviewees (graduates and nongraduates) reported having participated in paid internships or receiving vocational training while students at MCIP. MCIP's career development program proved to be very effective in preparing students for future careers. Thirty-eight (65 percent) of the 58 interviewees who participated in internships or received vocational instruction at MCIP were employed in 1988 in fields related to the training they received at the school. The largest number of interviewees by far (28 people) received training and were subsequently employed (21 individuals) in secretarial positions. The second most common category of career development activities was health care. Nine of the 11 interviewees who participated in MCIP-sponsored internships in this area were employed in health care or dentistry in 1988. Most youths who went on to work in fields related to their career development activities at MCIP went on to receive additional training after leaving high school. For many like Rosalba, MCIP administered the postsecondary career development programs, as well.

THE PASSAGE FROM ADOLESCENCE TO ADULTHOOD

While attending MCIP in 1982 and 1983, three-fourths of study participants indicated that they hoped to enter professional careers, most of which required a college education. By 1988, few informants had been able to obtain the college education that they had desired. On the other hand, two-thirds of MCIP graduates and one-half of all informants had obtained some type of postsecondary education and virtually all were employed. One in five already was working in professional or managerial positions in 1988. Few had become trapped in the poverty in which most lived shortly after arriving in Washington. Although many expressed regrets that they had not been able to obtain more education, most were satisfied with their jobs and generally happy with what had happened in their lives since leaving high school.

Postsecondary Education

Basic data regarding postsecondary education were gathered for 146 (81 percent) of the 181 persons in the study population, and more extensive educational histories were collected in interviews with 112 persons. Half of the group (73 of 146) had completed a job training program, earned

Table 9.1. Educational Achievement After High School

Postsecondary Education	Males (N = 73)		Females (N = 73)		Total (N = 146)	
	No.	%	No.	%	No.	%
None	46	(64)	28	(38)	75	(51)
Completed job training program	16	(22)	31	(42)	47	(32)
1 or more years of college	6	(8)	7	(10)	13	(9)
Associate degree (AD)	2	(3)	5	(7)	7	(5)
AD plus at least 1 year of college	2	(3)	2	(3)	4	(3)

an associate degree, or finished at least one year of college. (See Table 9.1.)

Women were more likely to have received some type of postsecondary education than men (χ^2 = 7.8, p < .01, 1 degree of freedom [df]). This difference is primarily explained by the fact that nearly twice as many young women as men completed job training programs. Better-paying jobs held by women in this study (e.g., secretary, health care worker) all required some type of postsecondary schooling or job training. In contrast, better-paying jobs not requiring education or vocational training (e.g., chef, waiter, and construction worker) were almost exclusively held by men.

By far the most frequently utilized form of postsecondary education was the job training program. In addition to career development programs in which study participants were involved while in high school, 58 of 112 interviewees reported having enrolled in one or more job training programs offered by public schools and colleges, community organizations, private trade schools, corporate employers, and the military. Interviewees successfully completed 75 percent of these programs. By far the largest number of postsecondary job training programs (28) were in office management.

Eleven informants had earned associate degrees, including four individuals who were continuing their university studies. Nine of the eleven informants who had earned associate degrees had been introduced to their fields through internships arranged by MCIP.

By 1988, 12 percent of all interviewees and 20 percent of those who were high school graduates had earned at least one year of credits toward a bachelors degree. None, however, had graduated from a 4-year baccalaureate program. Although most study participants had indicated that they wanted to go to college while they were in high school, two

Table 9.2. Jobs Held by Study Participants in 1988[a]

Job Category	Male No.	Male %	Female No.	Female %	Total No.	Total %
Restaurant and food service	17	22	7	10	24	16
Clerical	1	1	22	31	23	16
Business	9	12	5	7	14	10
Other services	10	13	7	10	17	12
Medical and dental	3	4	10	14	13	9
Construction	12	16	0	0	12	8
Other labor	11	14	0	0	11	7
Other skilled labor	9	12	1	1	10	7
Domestic: child care and housekeeping	0	0	9	13	9	6
Commercial cleaning and maintenance	3	4	2	3	5	3
Community wokers	1	1	3	4	4	3
Housewife	—	—	3	4	3	2
Unemployed	0	0	1	1	1	1
Totals	76	99	70	98	146	100

[a]Percent total does not equal 100% due to rounding.

obstacles repeatedly prevented them from making progress toward this goal.

1. *Immigration status.* When informants graduated from MCIP and were ready to enter college, many had not yet become legal residents of the United States. Some informants explained that they were afraid that they would be deported if they tried to take college courses. Others said that, without residency papers, they would not be able to afford higher out-of-state tuition and did not qualify for student loans.

2. *The need to work.* The need to work interfered with the pursuit of a college education in at least two ways. First, most informants worked long hours while attending MCIP and after graduating. Because of this, some did not have sufficient time to devote to their studies. Second, because most informants had to work to support themselves and other members of their families, they could not afford the cost of tuition and lost wages.

Employment

Finding employment seldom was a problem for participants in this study. By 1988, most informants had advanced well beyond the entry-level jobs that they held when they first arrived (Table 9.2). Clerical and restaurant work were by far the most common categories of employment for study participants. For the many women who had learned skills such as word processing and bookkeeping at MCIP or in postsecondary training programs, clerical work was perceived as providing adequate employment for the present and possibilities for career mobility for the future. For many men who had little education, restaurant work provided the chance for a limited amount of upward mobility, and incomes well above the poverty line. Nevertheless, most who worked in this field wished that they had jobs that required a formal education. They knew that they already had advanced as far as they could go in their current field. Most wished to have jobs where they would be respected for what they knew, rather than merely for how hard they worked, or for their "good attitude." The majority of study participants who had learned job skills at MCIP and elsewhere generally were able to find such jobs.

Interviewees seldom mentioned a lack of money as having been a major problem since leaving high school. Those who had not developed job skills, however, frequently reported that they could not find "good jobs." As discussed above, what was considered a "good job" was not defined solely by the wages that were paid.

Education and job skills were particularly important for women seeking employment in jobs with adequate salaries. Both men and women, however, considered education and vocational skills to be indispensable for job security. Those without these skills had only their hard work and a compliant attitude to rely on to please their bosses. Indeed, in the first years after arriving in Washington, most study participants had little alternative but to work very hard for little pay to survive.

Challenges and Hopes

By 1988, most study participants had become permanent residents of the United States or were applying for residency through the amnesty provision of the 1986 immigration law. Permanent residency was perceived as opening the door to better jobs, more security, and protection from exploitation. After years of working harder than others to survive, most were looking forward to taking the next step toward occupational mobility and economic security. For some who had not qualified for legal residency by 1988, however, "making it" in the United States by studying and working hard appeared increasingly unrealistic.

The disillusionment of some was aptly expressed in comments by Luis, an MCIP dropout from El Salvador. In 1988 he discussed how he had gotten involved while in high school with "friends who were not really my friends." He had no relatives present in Washington, and had been solely responsible for supporting himself since he arrived in Washington in 1980. One positive experience that he recalled from his days at the school was an internship that the school arranged for him at an auto parts store. Working there made him feel that he could do something right; it gave him a sense of competence. Unfortunately, when he dropped out of school, his internship ended. Since then, Luis had been working as a house painter. When asked about his hopes for the future, Luis was not very optimistic.

> I hope to survive. One of my biggest problems is not having confidence in myself. To make it in this country, you have to have a good education. You need a good job, and you need to have somebody there for you, to help you when you need it. A lot of us Latinos have problems with the same things: money and [immigration] papers. Maybe with the new [1986 immigration] law, the problem with the papers will be taken care of. But for people who came after me [after 1981, the cutoff date for the amnesty provision of the law]—they are going to be living at the same time in this country and in another. That is something that can really screw you up; it can totally confuse you.

Most of the refugee youths in this study had "become legal," gotten some education and vocational training, and gained a measure of economic security. Legal residents like Luis, who had not been able to get an education, will continue to rely on their hard work, "good attitude," and skills learned on the job. For many of the Central American refugees who have not become eligible for legal residency, however, even these attributes may ultimately be of little value.

When asked about their hopes for the future, most informants in this study indicated a desire to settle in, settle down and get ahead. In contrast to the wishes they had expressed shortly after arriving in Washington in the early 1980s, few hoped to return to live in their countries. By 1988, their hopes closely conformed to very traditional North American aspirations. For example, the hopes most commonly mentioned by interviewees were: to develop a future professional career (32 percent), have a family (21), earn a professional degree (18), go into business (17), enter any "good" career (17), get more education (14), and own a home (12).

When informants were asked if they had experienced any major disappointments since leaving high school, 66 of 112 interviewees stated that they had. The most common response by far (40 individuals) related to the inability to continue with their schooling. The next most frequently cited disappointments were: marital problems (10 informants), problems with immigration status (7), death in the family (9), inability to find a "good job" (6), illness or injury (4), and economic difficulties (3).

Interviewees also were asked in 1988 to name the greatest challenges that they and other Hispanic young adults had faced as they made the transition from adolescence to adulthood. One of the most frequently cited challenges (26 persons) was the need for young Washington, D.C. Latinos to set goals and then to work steadily to achieve them. Indeed, this was perhaps the most salient message communicated to students at MCIP. Other frequently mentioned challenges were: drug and alcohol abuse (33 individuals), getting an education (23), learning English (17), negative peer pressure (16), finding a good job (13), getting used to life in the United States (10), immigration problems (9), discrimination against them as foreigners (7), and loneliness (5).

Many of these problems and challenges described by informants were summarized well by Vicente, an exceptionally articulate and informed observer of street life. Vicente was one of several interviewees who had experienced serious problems related to drugs or immoderate alcohol consumption.[2] Although he had been a good student, had graduated from MCIP, and had subsequently held responsible jobs, Vicente believed that many of his problems were the result of what happened to him when he first came to the United States from Central America in 1981 at the age of 15. Vicente, his parents, and his brother were apprehended and jailed for entering the country illegally. Although his father was a Salvadorean government official who was seeking refuge for himself and his family because of an assassination attempt, Vicente and his family continued to experience serious problems with their immigration status. This made him bitter, and the insecurity of not knowing whether he would be deported made it difficult for him to plan for his future. When interviewed in 1988, he had exhausted his court appeals and was about to be deported. He had these comments about the attraction of the drug scene for youths like himself:

> [Drugs are] the worst. But at the time you live through it, they don't seem too bad; I mean, it's fun! Everything is Party! Party! Party! Party all the time. But you have to realize that you cannot live like that. If that were life, the whole world would be screwed up. But when the world is screwed up for you already anyway, it looks pretty good.

CONCLUSION

When first contacted in 1982 and 1983, the youths in this study had recently arrived in Washington, D.C., most as refugees from the political

---

[2]One of the original 181 Hispanic participants in the 1982 study had died of a drug overdose.

and economic turmoil of Central America. Seeing much danger and little hope for the future in the countries where they were born, they made the passage from their native countries to the capital city of the United States. In doing so, most came with little money and no knowledge of the English language or of urban North American culture. Indeed, many who were raised in rural areas had little knowledge of urban life in their own countries. When they arrived in Washington, they were confronted with the necessity of making sense of their new environment and establishing the niche they would occupy within it. They were compelled to reconstruct a coherent image of themselves in the context of their new society.

MCIP, the school attended by all study participants, was specifically designed to overcome the linguistic, cultural, and economic barriers that could prevent recent immigrant and refugee youths from effective participation in U.S. society. Most of the school's staff were bilingual and sensitive to the many pressing needs of the students and their families. MCIP facilitated its students' structural integration into the economic and social system of America through internships and job training programs. It promoted structural integration but did not rush cultural assimilation. MCIP communicated to its students the message that participation in the U.S. economic and social systems did not require abandoning their own cultures and languages. Acculturation pressures were mitigated through the multicultural orientation of the school's curriculum and extracurricular activities. Culture shock and other adjustment difficulties were addressed through counseling services.

Equally important as these core components of the MCIP program was the community that formed around the school itself. That community became a positive influence in the lives of many of these refugee youths. The MCIP community provided a viable social and cultural framework within which most of these young people were able to reconstruct a coherent image of themselves in their new society. The confidence they gained and support they found within the MCIP environment enabled most to overcome the many serious stressors they encountered in their dramatic passages from Latin America to Washington, D.C., from refugee to immigrant minority, and from adolescence to adulthood. The school culture emphasized respect for self and others and tolerance for cultural differences, and helped foster students' hopes that they could be successful in their new society while assisting them in their common purpose of acquiring the knowledge and skills that would enable them to do so. Along with other Hispanic community organizations in Washington, MCIP helped create a social environment which, for many, provided the security and stability of a surrogate family. In short, MCIP functioned as a mediating structure (Berger, 1976;

Berger and Neuhaus, 1981)—a community-based institution with which these refugee youths strongly identified, and within which they acquired both the skills and values that would enable them to become competent participants in their new society. This is illustrated by the 1988 comments of Edgar and Felipe, two successful MCIP graduates.

In 1988, Edgar described how MCIP and a church-sponsored Hispanic youth group enabled him to avoid becoming trapped in a pattern of self-destructive behavior.

> A lot of the kids that come here—they don't have nobody. They don't have no family. But that's not a reason not to do something with your life. I know a lot of people who lived by themselves—working and going to school, working and going to school. They can do it. There are guys who wish there was somebody to push them to do something—to improve their lives. Somebody out there to say, "Hey! I'm here! I'm here to help you one way or another. What can I do for you?" A lot of kids just don't have that somebody out there. I'm pretty sure that that's the way it is with 90 percent of the people.
>
> There are a lot of people out there who you can talk to, but not a lot of people you can trust. . . . My family, the school, and the youth group: that's how I've been able to learn how to be myself, to know who I am, and where I'm going.

By 1988, Edgar had earned an associate degree in medical technology and was employed in a hospital. He was continuing his studies at a local college in pursuit of a prelaw degree.

As discussed above, Felipe was studying nursing in 1988 and was deeply involved in community development work in the Hispanic community. He succinctly summarizes the different ways in which MCIP served him.

> One of the best things that has happened to me, I think, is the experience that I had at MCIP. I'm talking about all the things that I learned. I learned about the career of nursing—what it's like, and what you have to do to get in. But it is not just that [career development], or academics, but what I learned as a human being—as a person. In that aspect I think that MCIP has helped me to better relate to everything here. Even though I didn't have anyone like family to advise me, I had MCIP counselors who were great, who I will never forget. They were the only source that I had then—to come over and talk. I didn't have parents. They were the only ears that I had to listen to me. They were the only ones who could try to understand me, about the things that I did and I didn't like about this

society. At the same time, I learned to relate not only to Hispanics, but to Vietnamese, Chinese, Africans, [and] people from the Middle East. I think that the multicultural way has been really helpful to me because now I can see the good in everyone.

MCIP was not the only institutional resource available to these refugee youths while they were in high school. Latino community organizations also were important sources of institutional support for many. Together, the school and community organizations formed a culturally and geographically accessible network of institutions within which these youths received a variety of necessary services, and within which they developed the practical skills and values that facilitated their successful participation in U.S. society. Together, they formed a network of mediating structures that functioned in a manner similar to the settlement houses of previous decades (Addams, 1981). They provided a wide range of educational and social services (e.g., academic instruction, vocational training, counseling services, recreational activities, artistic expression) in familiar and culturally appropriate settings. Most youths learned how to become competent participants in their new society through their involvement in these instrumentally and emotionally rewarding activities. At the cultural level, the communication of values and norms through membership in the community that was centered around the school and community organizations was, in many ways, as valuable as the specific services that these institutions delivered.

Despite its many successes, MCIP could not guarantee the successful adaptation of all students. In addition to the unique problems that many had as de facto refugees, study participants also had to confront the same array of challenges as other poor, minority youths growing up in U.S. cities. Nonetheless, the predominant pattern of successful adaptation described here suggests that schools like MCIP not only can be effective in educating individual refugee youths, but may also play a key role in helping refugees successfully confront other problems associated with resettlement.

ACKNOWLEDGMENTS

Some of the field research was conducted by Ms. Marvette Perez, research assistant at the Catholic University of America. The research was supported by a grant from the Rockefeller Foundation. The content of this chapter is the sole responsibility of the author.

REFERENCES

Addams, J. (1981). *Twenty Years at Hull House.* New York: New American Library.

Berger, P. (1976). In praise of particularity: The concept of mediating structures. *Review of Politics, 38,* 399–410.

Berger, P., and Neuhaus, R. (1981). *To Empower People: The Role of Mediating Structures in Public Policy.* Washington, D.C.: American Enterprise Institute.

Cohen, L. M. (1979). *Culture, Disease, and Stress among Latino Immigrants.* Washington, D.C.: Research Institute on Immigration and Ethnic Studies, Smithsonian Institution.

Cohen, L. M. (1980). Stress and coping among Latin American women immigrants. In G. V. Coelho and P. I. Ahmed (eds.), *Uprooting and Development: Dilemmas of Coping with Modernization.* New York: Plenum.

Fine, M. (1986). Why urban adolescents drop into and out of public high school. *Teacher's College Record, 87,* 393–409.

Grier, E., and Grier, G. (1988). *People: Low-Income Adults of Working Age in Washington, D.C.* Washington, D.C.: Greater Washington Research Center.

Inda, C. (1981). *Perfil de la Comunidad Salvadoreña en Washington, D.C.* Washington, D.C.: D.C. Community Humanities Council.

Opportunities Industrialization Centers of America (1982). *The Career Intern Program: A Serious Solution to Youth Unemployment.* Philadelphia: Opportunities Industrialization Centers of America.

Singh, V., McGivern, E., and D'Emilio, T. (1981). *A Socioeconomic Needs Assessment Study Within the Hispanic Community in the Washington, D.C. Metropolitan Area.* Washington, D.C.: Spanish Education Development Center.

10 Toward the Development of Preventive Interventions for Youth Traumatized by War and Refugee Flight

CAROLYN L. WILLIAMS, Ph.D.

Half of the world's refugees are children under the age of 18 years (Dewey, 1988). For too many of these children, the trauma of the refugee experience is compounded by malnutrition, violence and torture, war injuries, and the loss of parents or other close relatives. The special needs of youthful refugees are beginning to be recognized, as evidenced by books like this; a recent historical, psychological, and legal study of unaccompanied children (Ressler, Boothby, and Steinbock, 1988); and the June 1988 special issue on children of *Refugees*, a publication of the United Nations High Comission for Refugees (UNHCR). In fact, the UNHCR sees one of its primary purposes being the provision of care to children (Dewey, 1988). While providing for children's physical and survival needs, attention is also being directed to refugee children's psychological, emotional, and educational needs (Crisp, 1988; Gerety, 1988; Mougne and Deya, 1988; Nettleton, 1988; Ressler et al., 1988). Despite the increasing interest in refugee children and the promotion of their mental health, very few, if any, true primary prevention programs exist for them. This chapter examines reasons for the scarcity of these programs, why they are needed, and the steps necessary for their development.

REFUGEE MENTAL HEALTH AND THE PRIMARY PREVENTION OF PSYCHOPATHOLOGY

Two primary sources of research are available to aid in the development of programs to alleviate or lessen the psychological and emotional

Portions of this chapter were taken from a 1987 report prepared for the National Institute of Mental Health's Refugee Assistance Program—Mental Health Technical Assistance Center of the University of Minnesota (contract no. 278-85-0024 CH). The opinions expressed herein are those of the author and do not necessarily reflect the official position of the NIMH or the U.S. Department of Health and Human Services.

trauma experienced by refugee children: work on the refugee experience and refugee mental health (e.g., Owan, 1985a; Ressler et al., 1988; Stein, 1981a,b, 1986; Williams, 1987a; Williams and Westermeyer, 1986) and the literature on the primary prevention of psychopathology (e.g., Caplan, 1964; Edelstein and Michelson, 1986; Felner et al., 1983; Klein and Goldston, 1977). Unfortunately, progress in both fields has been hampered in the past for several reasons. The primary prevention field has been impeded by vague definitions and concepts (Spaulding and Balch, 1983). Difficulties inherent in refugee research include the need for a multidisciplinary perspective; a tendency to view each refugee movement as isolated, deviant, and nonrecurring; and the constant reinventing of the wheel with each new refugee exodus (Ressler et al., 1988; Stein, 1981a,b, 1986).

A major step toward compiling information about the special needs of children who were without parents or other care-givers because of refugee movements and other disasters was taken when the Norwegian Save the Children organization (Redd Barna) encouraged a study about unaccompanied children (Ressler et al., 1988). This project was supported by grants from the Ford Foundation, Norwegian Save the Children, UNHCR, United Nations Childrens Fund (UNICEF), Save the Children Federation, Diakonisches Werk, and International Union of Child Welfare (IUCW). A series of recommendations, including suggestions for preparedness and prevention, assistance, and interim and permanent placements, were developed and endorsed by UNICEF and the UNHCR (Ressler et al., 1988).

Other steps addressing refugee mental health needs were taken three years ago in the United States when the National Institute of Mental Health (NIMH), in collaboration with the Office of Refugee Resettlement (ORR), implemented the Refugee Assistance Program: Mental Health (RAP) and funded the University of Minnesota as the Technical Assistance Center (TAC) for RAP. One of the major tasks of the multidisciplinary TAC was to produce materials on the refugee experience that would be used by states in their efforts to upgrade mental health services and mainstream mental health care for refugees resettled in the United States. Many of the TAC documents and materials were distributed beyond the 12 funded RAP states and should improve the problems in the refugee field noted by Stein (1981a,b, 1986). Three reports funded by TAC (Berry, 1988; Williams, 1987b, 1989) and a TAC training videotape for mental health professionals (Williams, Garcia-Peltoniemi, and Ben-Porath, 1988) integrate the research on refugee mental health with the primary prevention of psychopathology literature. Other TAC reports containing useful information for prevention program planners summarized the psychosocial stressors of the refugee experience (Ben-

Porath, 1987) and the common forms of psychopathology in refugees (Garcia-Peltoniemi, 1987).

Williams (1987b, 1989) identified a major impediment to the development of prevention programs for refugees that paralleled the definitional problems characterizing the general field of the prevention of mental disorders. In the early days of the community mental health movement, some advocates suggested that almost all aspects of human behavior and social conditions were within their domain. This tendency was labeled "boundarylessness and boundary busting" (Dinitz and Beran, 1971, p. 99). Zax and Cowen (1976, p. 479) pointed out that "virtually anything done to improve man's lot can also be viewed as primary mental health prevention." Boundarylessness is apparent in refugee mental health when resettlement and social services are described as ways to improve the mental health of refugees. However, simply labeling a program as primary prevention does not mean that it will reduce the number of mental health cases; instead, it may have disappointing results that will be used to justify the termination of scarce resources. In addition, without agreement on the scope of prevention programs, "discussants will often be examining several different phenomena while thinking they are focusing on one" (Lamb and Zusman, 1979, p. 12). Boundarylessness also increases the probability of reliance on ideology rather than empirically tested methods, and increases the likelihood of promising better results than what is actually possible (Spaulding and Balch, 1983).

Cowen (1977, 1982, 1985) concluded that because of the lack of an operational definition of prevention programs and prevention research, many diverse endeavors were inaccurately called prevention, undercutting the field's most important potential contribution, that of presenting alternatives to current mental health practices. Problems with the all-inclusiveness of past definitions of prevention were also noted in an NIMH publication on Southeast Asian mental health (Silverman, 1985). The definitional problems occurred partly because the terms "prevention" and "promotion" were borrowed from the public health field and do not translate readily into the mental health field. In public health, prevention is almost always used in the context of illness, whereas mental health practitioners deal not only with individuals with diagnosable mental illness but also with those who are not ill but want help with disturbing interpersonal problems and distresses of daily living (Lamb and Zusman, 1979) and with victims of stress, powerlessness, and exploitation (Albee, 1979, 1986). As described above, some mental health practitioners believe that general societal problems come within their purview and that social change and redistribution of power are needed to reduce psychopathology (Albee, 1979, 1986).

Perhaps these definitional issues, along with the constant reinventing of the wheel in refugee mental health, explain the lack of effective primary prevention programs for refugee children, despite opportunities in prevention at three levels: international, national, and local. Effective primary prevention for refugee children could be developed at the international policy level (i.e., by policies that decrease the likelihood of refugee movements and wars or through policies to prevent the separation of children from their families during these emergencies (Ressler et al., 1988); at the national policy level (e.g., by national resettlement policies that promote cluster resettlement or the resettlement of families and other natural support systems in the same location); or at the local level in resettlement countries (i.e., where most Western-trained mental health professionals are able to develop programs). Three steps will be described to facilitate development of primary prevention programs at these levels.

Step 1: Clarifying the Definitions of Prevention

Prevention efforts traditionally are classified as primary, secondary, or tertiary. Table 10.1 presents definitions from the literature.

Some have argued that only primary prevention should be considered synonymous with prevention, since secondary and tertiary prevention are actually treatment and rehabilitation (Goldston, 1986a,b). However, as described by Goldston (1986a,b), the field developed with this confusion of terms.

Primary Prevention: Specific Protection. Primary prevention offers the greatest possibility for a new approach to mental health problems (Silverman, 1985). Primary prevention activities typically represent either specific protection or health promotion. *Specific protection* involves using a highly specific procedure that is effective in preventing one disorder, but does not appear effective in preventing any other disorder (Bloom, 1979). Public health programs, such as providing immunization for smallpox or destroying the mosquito that carries malaria, are examples of specific protection in disease prevention. Specific protection procedures are effective for some mental disorders, particularly those arising from certain infectious or genetic processes; nutritional deficiencies; physical injuries; general systemic diseases; and environmental agents like poisons, chemicals, toxic gases, and licit or illicit drug overdoses (Bloom, 1979). For example, pellagra, a chronic disease caused by a deficiency of niacin in the diet, accounted for a significant percentage of the admissions to psychiatric facilities in the southern United States during the last century. Dietary improvements now prevent the occur-

Table 10.1. Definitions of Prevention Terms

Primary Prevention
Lowers the rate (i.e., incidence) of new emotional disorders in a population
Counteracts irritants before they exact a toll
Builds health and resources in people from the start
Performed in a mass-oriented way before trouble starts
Prevents diseases from ever occurring
Lowers the rate of new cases of mental disorder in a population over a certain
   period (i.e., incidence) by counteracting harmful forces before they have a
   chance to produce illness
Uses techniques that seek to reduce the prevalence (i.e., total number of
   cases) of a disorder by reducing its incidence
Removes causes, known or hypothesized, of disease or disorders

Secondary Prevention
Enables a person to regain his or her normal level of functioning and prevents
   further development of illness after its occurrence
Uses techniques that seek to reduce the prevalence of a disorder by reducing
   its duration
Focuses on early detection and prompt treatment to prevent disorders from
   becoming more serious
Halts the progression of existing diseases

Tertiary Prevention
Reduces the severity, discomfort, or disability associated with any disorder
Rehabilitates the individual
Prevents or reverses the aftereffects of illness (i.e., disability)
Focuses on rehabilitation of the individual during or following illness along
   pathways (e.g., jobs, housing, training) that lead to independent living and
   minimize permanent disability

Source: From Williams, C. L., and Westermeyer, J. (eds.). (1986). *Refugee Mental Health in Resettlement Countries.* Washington, D.C.: Hemisphere.

rence of this disease in developed countries. However, refugees often come from parts of the world without adequate nutrition, general health care, or even sanitary and healthy environments. Mental health and public health officials working solely in this country may not be aware of some of these preventable mental disorders and the specific protection procedures available.

Consultation with public health professionals familiar with the conditions in the refugees' home countries is essential to implement appropriate specific protection procedures. Particular attention should be paid to nutritional disorders that may result from the unfamiliar foods and preparation methods, and greater expense of some foods in the host country; harmful folk remedies; improper use of medications or other drugs; and endemic infectious diseases or other illnesses in the home country that may lead to mental disorders.

Primary Prevention: Health Promotion. Health promotion is the other major classification for primary prevention programs. These programs represent a variety of nonspecific practices that may improve health in general and may actually prevent some behavior disorders (Bloom, 1979). The rationale for *health promotion* is to enhance the individual's (or *host*'s, to use an epidemiological term) ability to resist disease, even when the disease agents are not known or are beyond control (Eisenberg, 1981). Mental health promotion techniques are generally less well-known than specific protection strategies and thought to involve a greater social, as well as economic, cost (Bloom, 1979). There are also fewer empirical demonstrations of the effectiveness of mental health promotion programs. Unfortunately, full-scale public mental health programs have been initiated in the past without adequate attention to their possible iatrogenic consequences or other contraindications (Arnhoff, 1975; Spaulding and Balch, 1983; Westermeyer, 1987). Lorion (1986) provides additional examples of prevention interventions with serious negative effects like McCord's (1978) long-term follow-up of a classic prevention effort aimed at delinquency-prone adolescents. McCord (1978) demonstrated that adolescents who were identified in the 1950s as delinquency-prone and randomly assigned to a prevention-oriented counseling program had a worse outcome in adulthood than the no-treatment control group! Because of this, an empirical evaluation of program effectiveness is essential to avoid possible ill effects, as well as to serve local populations better (Price and Smith, 1985).

Given the trauma experienced by refugees, they represent a "natural experiment" for testing the efficacy of health promotion programs designed to reduce the harmful effects of stressful experiences. Programs developed and demonstrated to be effective for refugees also may be effective for other populations, such as ethnic and racial minorities, who often share similar circumstances (e.g., cultural differences, marginal social status, and problems of racism and poverty). This adds to the attractiveness of funding prevention programs for refugees, particularly in the light of Owan's (1985b) description of the changing demographics that are making the United States a nation of minorities.

Previous work strongly suggests that the development of prevention programs for refugee children will be feasible only if the prominent definitional issues described above are taken into account by planners. As Owan (1985b) recommended, a primary prevention program for refugee children must meet Cowen's (1982, p. 132) three structural requirements:

1. It must be group—or mass—rather than individual-oriented (even though some of its activities may involve individual contacts).

2. It must have a before-the-fact quality, that is, it must be targeted to groups not yet experiencing significant maladjustment (even though they may, because of their life situations or recent experiences, be at risk for such outcomes).

3. It must be intentional, that is, it must rest on a solid knowledge-base, suggesting that the program holds potential for either improving psychological health or preventing maladaptation.

Step 2: Identifying Mental Health Problems of Refugee Children

With these definitional issues in mind, we can now turn to a discussion of some of the common mental health issues and problems facing refugee children. Unfortunately, little attention has been directed to refugee children (with the exception of the study on unaccompanied children by Ressler et al., 1988), and so some of this discussion is extracted from the adult literature. Children experience the same psychosocial stages of the refugee experience as identified for adults (Ben-Porath, 1987), yet the meaning of these stages for children remains to be described. During the early stages of the refugee movement (i.e., preflight chaos and the period of flight), children, like the adults around them, often are in grave physical danger. These early stages have important implications for later prevention program development.

Smyke (1988) describes some of the emotions and experiences children have during the early stages of refugee flight. Frequently they witness their parents' mounting anxieties and sense of powerlessness. The children's confidence in their parents' ability to manage their world is gravely shaken. Perhaps they have witnessed violence and killing, or have been separated from their parents, who may choose to remain behind to fight, or may be imprisoned, or may be dead. Parents may intentionally avoid telling the children what their plans are for fear the children will give away the plans, causing great harm to the family. In these circumstances, children will make up their own explanations, which often involves taking on a sense of responsibility and guilt about what has happened. Smyke (1988, p. 22) gives an example of this with a quote from one little Pakistani girl, the victim of a bomb attack: "Oh, what have we done now that they need to bomb us again?"

In addition to the emotional trauma of the flight, malnutrition, illnesses, and injuries are quite common. In some instances parents have accidentally suffocated infants or young children when they cry out and risk betraying the family to the enemy. As Carlin (1986) points out, the age of the child experiencing these difficulties is important in relation to the developmental tasks that are interrupted by these harmful experiences.

By the time the family, if it is able to remain intact, reaches the safety of the refugee camp, parents may be so overburdened with their own losses, adjustment to refugee status, and attending to the basic survival needs of the family that they are unable to address the emotional needs of their children. Thus, it is in refugee camps where prevention programming for children and their families must begin. And, as Ressler et al. (1988) indicate, programs for refugee children must be equally accessible to those with parents and those unaccompanied. Risks are high that unaccompanied children will not receive adequate services if they are not targeted, and there is the converse problem of parents abandoning children if unaccompanied status is perceived as affording the children greater benefits and services in the camp.

In addition to specific protection programs for nutritional, genetic, and systemic diseases, mental health promotion programs should be developed in refugee camps. These prevention efforts must be made in the context of what precedes the refugee flight. Mental health professionals must be educated about these events to develop effective prevention programs. Fortunately, there are good summaries of the antecedent stressors and theories about refugee behavior (e.g., Ben-Porath, 1987; Stein, 1981a,b, 1986).

During final resettlement, two sources of psychosocial stress have direct relevance for children: family stressors and cultural barriers (Ben-Porath, 1987). It has been widely documented across many refugee movements that children tend to acculturate faster than do adults, which leads to intergenerational conflicts. Another major source of difficulty for refugee adjustment is when there are great cultural differences between the host and home countries, with the accompanying acculturative stress (Berry, 1988).

Mental disorders, particularly the anxiety and depressive disorders, have been shown to have a higher prevalence among adult refugees compared to the general population (Garcia-Peltoniemi, 1987; Westermeyer, 1986). Case reports of refugee children and adolescents also suggest a higher prevalence of mental disorders in refugee children compared to the general population (Harding and Looney, 1986; Nettleton, 1988; Szaporcznik, Cohen, and Hernandez, 1985; Williams and Westermeyer, 1983). However, we are less clear about the specific mental disorders common in refugee children, and it may well be that the prevalence of various disorders may be dependent on the cultural, historical, and political aspects of the particular refugee exodus. For example, the Mariel Cuban exodus had an abundance of unaccompanied adolescents with a history of acting-out problems (Szapocznik et al., 1985). Media reports also indicate that many Amerasian youth in Vietnam may have been "street children," which also suggests a greater prevalence of acting-out problems. On the other hand, Cambodian youth frequently endured malnutrition, torture, and injuries, suggesting a higher prevalence of cognitive impairments and learning difficulties in that group. Ressler et al. (1988) suggest age-dependent differences in children's symptoms (e.g., infants and toddlers may exhibit intense crying, food refusals, digestive upsets, and sleeping problems; whereas adolescents may exhibit depressed mood, withdrawal, aggressive behaviors, and somatic reactions including headaches and stomach aches).

It is evident that for any refugee exodus, a needs assessment of the mental health of the children is required. The above overview suggests areas to investigate. Yet it is likely, based on past experience, that the children in each exodus will have had slightly different experiences that will necessitate different types of programs. Such a needs assessment should be carried out early in the refugee movement, preferably in the camps of first asylum. Preflight and flight experiences, family status, nutritional and physical health needs, age of the children, and observations of current behavior should be included. Ressler et al. (1988) provide valuable insights about how programs must vary to meet developmental and other needs of refugee children.

Step 3: Integrating Prevention and Refugee Mental Health Programs for Children

Two models are available to guide efforts for prevention program development for refugee children (Williams, 1989). Bloom's (1982, p. 385) stressful life events is one such model:

1. Identify a stressful life event, or set of such events, that appear to have undesirable consequences. Develop procedures for reliably identifying persons who have undergone or who are undergoing those stressful experiences.

2. By traditional epidemiological and laboratory methods, study the consequences of those events and develop hypotheses related to how one might go about reducing or eliminating their negative consequences.

3. Mount and evaluate experimental preventive intervention programs based on these hypotheses.

Refugee children, as described above, undergo a series of negative life events and these children are relatively easy to identify (condition 1 of Bloom's model). Refugee mental health research suggests hypotheses about how to reduce some of the negative consequences of the experience (condition 2). For example, specific protection procedures to eliminate the harmful effects of nutritional and other likely disorders of refugee children are a possibility. Mental health promotion programs also are possible to develop (e.g., focusing on intergenerational conflict or the cultural barriers common at final resettlement). It is condition 3, evaluation, that currently is lacking.

One other model that can guide efforts in program development for refugee children is Albee's (1982, p. 1,046) prevention equation:

$$\text{Incidence} = \frac{\text{Organic factors} + \text{Stress}}{\text{Coping skills} + \text{Self-esteem} + \text{Support groups}}$$

An effective primary prevention program could reduce the incidence of a disorder (or the left side of the equation) either by decreasing the numerator or increasing the denominator. Preventive efforts designed to lower organic factors or stress or increase coping skills, self-esteem, or support groups should lower incidence. This formula demonstrates the multicausal nature of the incidence of psychopathology, which requires multiple levels of intervention.

Work with child populations in the United States suggests other possible prevention programs for refugees. Programs being examined empirically include providing adequate nutrition, mitigating the effects of acute loss through social support and other procedures, providing good prenatal care, improving schooling and child-rearing practices, developing coping skills of individuals at risk for problems, bolstering social networks, family planning, and genetic counseling (see Albee, 1982; Bloom, 1979, 1982; Cowen, 1977, 1985; Edelstein and Michelson, 1986; Eisenberg, 1981; Felner et al., 1983; Levine and Perkins, 1987; Munoz, 1976 for descriptions of these types of interventions). Many of these examples offer both specific protection against certain diseases and general health promotion. For example, providing adequate nutrition not only will prevent specific diseases like pellagra, but also will enhance the individual's ability to resist other disorders. Of course, it remains a challenge for prevention practitioners to provide these programs in a culturally sensitive and acceptable manner.

EXAMPLES OF PREVENTION PROGRAMS FOR REFUGEE CHILDREN IN CAMPS

A program in a Khmer refugee camp at Phanat Nikhom (Thailand) entitled "Preparation for American Secondary Schools" is an example of cultural preparation to smooth the transition for refugee adolescents and their parents (Munnell, 1985). Since many Khmer have little or no experience with formal education, this program introduces the American school system to the refugees. One part of the program deals specifically with parental involvement with their child's education, since the parental role in the United States is so different from what is expected in Asia. Although this is a good example of a preventive strategy, Munnell (1985) presented no evaluation information upon which to judge the program's utility.

Past mental health consultation in refugee camps in the United States illustrated the necessity of studying each group separately, rather than having one generic program for refugee children. After completing a needs assessment of the Vietnamese refugee children placed at Camp Pendleton in California, Harding and Looney (1986) and their colleagues offered a number of primary prevention suggestions including providing toys and athletic equipment; establishing centers to provide infant care, preschool programs, school programs, and adolescent activities within the camp; establishing central obstetrical and pediatric care; placing families as quickly as possible; maintaining the integrity of large families when resettling; and keeping any unaccompanied minors with "unofficial foster families," rather than separating them from the adults in the camp and placing them with American families.

Some similar programs were established for the Mariel Cuban adolescents in their refugee camps. However, a big difference occurred with the segregation of the minors from the rest of the camp population. For, unlike the Vietnamese adult camp population which consisted mostly of families, many of the Cubans were single adult men, including a few dangerous criminals. Minors were separated from the rest of the camp because of a concern for their safety (Szapocznik et al., 1985).

Unfortunately, the suggestions of the mental health consultants at Camp Pendleton were not heeded and the unaccompanied minors were separated from the rest of the camp, thus precluding an evaluation of the primary prevention intervention. The unaccompanied minors compound came to resemble a psychiatric facility (Harding and Looney, 1977). Reports indicated some problems with placing children in foster homes that were culturally dissimilar (e.g., Mortland and Egan, 1987; Ressler et al., 1988; Williams and Westermeyer, 1983). Particular problems occurred when the unaccompanied minors' natural parents arrived after the children had lived for many years in an American home, a problem documented in earlier refugee movements (Ressler et al., 1988). At the very least, more preparation is needed for American foster families (Mortland and Egan, 1987).

EXAMPLE OF A MENTAL HEALTH PROMOTION PROGRAM
FOR FINAL RESETTLEMENT

Most mental health professionals encounter refugees not in camps, but after they have resettled in communities in countries like the United States. They are unlikely to develop prevention programs at the international level (e.g., efforts to decrease war, violence, and refugee movements) as part of their professional role, and most do not participate in setting policies for refugee camps or national resettlement to promote mental health. It is at the local community level where most mental health professionals can begin primary prevention programs for refugee children. Duncan and Kang (1985) provide an example of a local-level mental health promotion program developed for Cambodian refugee children resettled by the Catholic Community Services in Tacoma, Washington. Although, like all other primary prevention programs for refugee children, it lacks the needed evaluation component, it illustrates nicely the potential for developing sound primary prevention programs for refugee children.

Duncan and Kang's (1985) program meets the definitional requirements for primary prevention: it follows the mental health promotion definition, rather than taking a specific protection approach. Cowen's (1982) structural requirements for primary prevention are met, in that the program is targeted to all unaccompanied Cambodian minors resettled in Tacoma, it has the required "before-the-fact quality" since the program is provided *before* the minor is identified as having a diagnosed mental disorder, and it is based on the knowledge that unaccompanied minors are an "at-risk" group (Ressler et al., 1988) and that culture and religious rituals often serve a protective function (Dubreuil and Wittkower, 1976) in times of grief and loss.

The program also follows Bloom's (1982) stressful life events model for prevention program development. As Duncan and Kang (1985) note, the Cambodian children endured extremely stressful life events including forced separations from families and friends, war and chaos in Cambodia, and possibly witnessing torture and killing of parents and others. Duncan and Kang (1985) hypothesized that the children's separation from families occurred under circumstances that prevented the children from resolving feelings of grief and loss. They noted that all the unaccompanied minors exhibited some sleep disturbances on arrival, with frequently disturbing dreams or nightmares of lost family members. In many cases children reported disturbing visits of spirits, often including one or both parents or grandparents. Duncan and Kang (1985, p. 3) further hypothesized "another massive loss—the loss of their culture or known world. By this, we mean that the cultural 'givens' of a child's world no longer operate successfully, leaving him or her without a rational world system to fall back onto."

Based on these hypotheses, Duncan and Kang (1985) developed a mental health promotion program designed to reduce the negative consequences of the Cambodian children's losses. The program included foster placements in ethnically similar homes, as has been suggested by others as optimal in many circumstances (Ressler et al., 1988). The main components of the program included the use of traditional Theravada Buddhist ceremonies and rituals to honor the dead, as well as consultation with Cambodian Buddhist spiritual leaders. For every unaccompanied minor, three ceremonies were used during their first year of resettlement: Ban Skol (a memorial for absent family members), Pratchun Ban (an annual family reunion of living and deceased relatives which is held yearly in Tacoma during late September or early October), and a religious observance for absent family members held in conjunction with Cambodian New Year in April.

The Ban Skol ceremony was performed by Buddhist monks in the child's foster home within a few months of the child's arrival in the United States, if possible. It was arranged jointly by the foster family and agency personnel and was performed specifically for the child's family members who were absent for whatever reason (dead, missing, or left behind in Cambodia). The foster family prepared special food to be offered to the monks and also a festive meal for all the family, guests, and agency staff in attendance. The child made a list of family he or she wished to remember or honor. The child, foster family, and agency staff sat in front of the monks, with all other guests behind, and everyone touching each other during the ceremony. The participants recited a chanted prayer, the monk burned the paper over a bowl and then poured water slowly over the ashes. This burning, symbolic of cremating the body of the deceased, was "particularly important for those children who saw their relatives' bodies left to rot or dumped in mass graves. Many children do not know what happened to their families but saw many other untended bodies and fear this fate for their own parents. Pouring the water and the ashes on the ground ensures that it will go to the loved ones even if they are not present. . . . The foster child who is the central figure in the ceremony receives help and support from the new foster family and their friends and from the caseworkers and thus the agency. . . . The children are often silent and withdrawn while participating in the ceremony or may be overcome with grief. They are generally consoled by family and guests and are especially drawn into the fun and laughter that follows during the meal" (Duncan and Kang, 1985, p. 8).

Anecdotal reports from the 47 Cambodian children who participated in this program suggest some grief resolution, decrease in sleep disturbances and spirit visits, and increased bonding with foster family members, after the Ban Skol ceremony (Duncan and Kang, 1985), although as the authors note, more systematic evaluation is needed. However, programs of this nature have great potential, demonstrating that the structural requirements for primary prevention can be met using culturally appropriate ceremonies that include participation from the mainstream American agency.

It is apparent that considerably more work is needed on the development of prevention programs for refugee youth. The need is great for this is a highly traumatized population, who must complete the developmental tasks of childhood in spite of their losses. The models for program development reviewed in this chapter emphasize the need for clarity in defining prevention programs, reliance on previous research on refugee behavior and refugee mental health, and an empirical verification of any program's outcome.

REFERENCES

Albee, G. W. (1979). Politics, power, prevention, and social change. *Clinical Psychologist, 33,* 12–13.

Albee, G. W. (1982). Preventing psychopathology and promoting human potential. *American Psychologist, 37,* 1043–1050.

Albee, G. W. (1986). Toward a just society: Lessons from observations on the primary prevention of psychopathology. *American Psychologist, 41,* 891–898.

Arnhoff, F. N. (1975). Social consequences of policy towards mental illness. *Science, 188,* 1277–1281.

Ben-Porath, Y. S. (1987). *Issues in the Psycho-social Adjustment of Refugees.* (Contract No. 278-85-0024 CH). Rockville, Md.: National Institute of Mental Health.

Berry, J. W. (1988). *Refugee Mental Health: Managing the Process of Acculturation for Problem Prevention.* (Contract No. 278-85-0024 CH). Rockville, Md.: National Institute of Mental Health.

Bloom, B. L. (1979). Prevention of mental disorders: Recent advances in theory and practice. *Community Mental Health Journal, 15,* 179–191.

Bloom, B. L. (1982). Epilogue. In S. M. Manson (ed.), *New Directions in Prevention Among American Indian and Alaska Native Communities,* pp. 377–394. Portland: Oregon Health Sciences University.

Caplan, G. (1964). *Principles of Preventive Psychiatry.* New York: Basic Books.

Carlin, J. E. (1986). Child and adolescent refugees: Psychiatric assessment and treatment. In C. L. Williams and J. Westermeyer (eds.), *Refugee Mental Health in Resettlement Countries,* pp. 131–139. New York: Hemisphere.

Cowen, E. L. (1977). Baby-steps toward primary prevention. *American Journal of Community Psychology, 5,* 1–22.

Cowen, E. L. (1982). Primary prevention research: Barriers, needs and opportunities. *Journal of Primary Prevention, 2,* 131–137.

Cowen, E. L. (1985). Primary prevention in mental health. *Social Policy, 15,* 11–17.

Crisp, J. (1988). Refugee children: Policy and practice. *Refugees, 54,* 19–20.

Dewey, A. E. (1988). Half the world's refugees. *Refugees, 54,* 16–18.

Dinitz, S., and Beran, N. (1971). Community mental health as a boundaryless and boundary-busting system. *Journal of Health and Social Behaviors, 12,* 99–107.

Dubreuil, G., and Wittkower, E. D. (1976). Primary prevention: A combined psychiatric-anthropological appraisal. In J. Westermeyer (ed.), *Anthropology and Mental Health: Setting a New Course,* pp. 31–48. New York: Pergamon.

Duncan, J., and Kang, S. (1985). Using Buddhist ritual activities as foundation for a mental health program for Cambodian children in foster care. Unpublished manuscript. (Available from J. Duncan, Lutheran Social Services, 6920 220th Street S.W., Mountlake Terrace, Wash. 98043.

Edelstein, B. A., and Michelson, L. (eds.). (1986). *Handbook of Prevention.* New York: Plenum.

Eisenberg, L. (1981). A research framework for evaluating the promotion of mental health and prevention of mental illness. *Public Health Reports, 96,* 3–19.

Felner, R. D., Jason, L. A., Moritsugu, J. N., and Farber, S. S. (eds.). (1983). *Preventive Psychology: Theory, Research, and Practice.* New York: Pergamon.

Garcia-Peltoniemi, R. (1987). *Psychopathology in Refugees.* (Contract No. 278-85-0024 CH). Rockville, Md.: National Institute of Mental Health.

Gerety, P. (1988). Philippines: Studying for the future. *Refugees, 54,* 27–28.

Goldston, S. E. (1986a). Primary prevention: Historical perspectives and a blueprint for action. *American Psychologist, 41,* 453–460.

Goldston, S. E. (1986b). The federal scene: Ten years later. In M. Kessler and S. E. Goldston (eds.), *A Decade of Progress in Primary Prevention,* pp. 363–388. Hanover, N.H.: University Press of New England.

Harding, R. K., and Looney, J. G. (1977). Problems of Southeast Asian children in a refugee camp. *American Journal of Psychiatry, 134,* 407–411.

Harding, R., and Looney, J. (1986). Mental health consultation in refugee camps. In C. L. Williams and J. Westermeyer (eds.), *Refugee Mental Health in Resettlement Countries,* pp. 205–216. New York: Hemisphere.

Klein, D. C., and Goldston, S. E. (eds.). (1977). *Primary Prevention: An Idea Whose Time Has Come* (Department of Health, Education, and Welfare Publication No. ADM 77-447). Washington, D.C.: U.S. Government Printing Office.

Lamb, R. H., and Zusman, J. (1979). Primary prevention in perspective. *American Journal of Psychiatry, 136,* 12–17.

Levine, M., and Perkins, D. V. (1987). *Principles of Community Psychology.* New York: Oxford University Press.

Lorion, R. P. (1986). Evaluating preventive interventions: Guidelines for the serious social change agent. In R. D. Felner, L. A. Jason, J. N. Moritsugu, and S. S. Farber (eds.), *Preventive Psychology: Theory, Research, and Practice*, pp. 251–268. New York: Pergamon.

McCord, J. (1978). A thirty-year follow-up of treatment effects. *American Psychologist, 35,* 1000–1011.

Mortland, C. A., and Egan, M. G. (1987). Vietnamese youth in American foster care. *Social Work, 32,* 240–245.

Mougne, C., and Deya, M. (1988). Zaire: Assisting Angolan children. *Refugees, 54,* 31–32.

Munnell, K. (1985). The youth and adult cultural orientation programs: How they can benefit each other. *Passage: A Journal of Refugee Education, 1,* 13–14.

Munoz, R. F. (1976). The primary prevention of psychological problems. *Community Mental Health Review, 1,* 4–15.

Nettleton, C. (1988). United Kingdom: Living in a new home. *Refugees, 54,* 29–30.

Owan, T. C. (ed.). (1985a). *Southeast Asian Mental Health: Treatment, Prevention, Services, Training, and Research* (Department of Health and Human Services Publication No. ADM 85-600553). Washington, D.C.: U.S. Government Printing Office.

Owan, T. C. (1985b). Southeast Asian mental health: Transition from treatment services to prevention—a new direction. In T. C. Owan (ed.), *Southeast Asian Mental Health: Treatment, Prevention, Services, Training, and Research* (Department of Health and Human Services Publication No. ADM 85-600553), pp. 141–167. Washington, D.C.: U.S. Government Printing Office.

Price, R. H., and Smith, S. S. (1985). *A Guide to Evaluating Prevention Programs in Mental Health* (Department of Health and Human Services Publication No. ADM 85-1365). Washington, D.C.: U.S. Government Printing Office.

Ressler, E. M., Boothby, N., and Steinbock, D. J. (1988). *Unaccompanied Children: Care and Protection in Wars, Natural Disasters, and Refugee Movements.* New York: Oxford University Press.

Silverman, M. M. (1985). Preventive intervention research: A new beginning. In T. C. Owan (ed.), *Southeast Asian Mental Health: Treatment, Prevention, Services, Training, and Research* (Department of Health and Human Services Publication No. ADM 85-600553), pp. 169–181. Washington, D.C.: U.S. Government Printing Office.

Smyke, P. (1988). Pakistan: Journey into exile. *Refugees, 54,* 21–22.

Spaulding, J., and Balch, P. (1983). A brief history of primary prevention in the twentieth century: 1908 to 1980. *American Journal of Community Psychology, 11,* 59–80.

Stein, B. N. (1981a). The refugee experience: Defining the parameters of a field of study. *International Migration Review, 15,* 320–330.

Stein, B. N. (1981b). Understanding the refugee experience: Foundations of a better resettlement system. *Journal of Refugee Resettlement, 1,* 62–71.

Stein, B. N. (1986). The experience of being a refugee: Insights from the research literature. In C. L. Williams and J. Westermeyer (eds.), *Refugee Mental Health in Resettlement Countries*, pp. 5–23. Washington, D.C.: Hemisphere.

Szapocznik, J., Cohen, R., and Hernandez, R. E. (1985). *Coping with Adolescent Refugees: The Mariel Boatlift*. New York: Praeger.

Westermeyer, J. (1986). Migration and psychopathology. In C. L. Williams and J. Westermeyer (eds.), *Refugee Mental Health in Resettlement Countries*, pp. 39–59. New York: Hemisphere.

Westermeyer, J. (1987). Public health and chronic mental illness. *American Journal of Public Health, 77,* 667–668.

Williams, C. L. (1987a). *An Annotated Bibliography on Refugee Mental Health* (Department of Health and Human Services Publication No. ADM 87-1517). Washington, D.C.: U.S. Government Printing Office.

Williams, C. L. (1987b). *Prevention Programs for Refugee Mental Health* (Contract No. 278-85-0024 CH). Rockville, Md.: National Institute of Mental Health.

Williams, C. L. (1989). Prevention program for refugees: An interface for mental health and public health. *Journal of Primary Prevention, 10,* 167–186.

Williams, C. L., Garcia-Peltoniemi, R. E., and Ben-Porath, Y. S. (1988). *Refugee Mental Health: The Importance of Primary Prevention* (videocassette) (Contract No. 278-85-0024 CH). Rockville, Md.: National Institute of Mental Health.

Williams, C. L., and Westermeyer, J. (1983). Psychiatric problems among adolescent Southeast Asian refugees. *Journal of Nervous and Mental Disease, 171,* 79–84.

Williams, C. L., and Westermeyer, J. (eds.). (1986). *Refugee Mental Health in Resettlement Countries*. Washington, D.C.: Hemisphere.

Zax, M., and Cowen, E. L. (1976). *Abnormal Psychology: Changing Conceptions,* 2nd ed. New York: Holt, Rinehart, & Winston.

Subject Index

Academic: achievement, 139; adjustment, 108–10, 112, 122; failure, 134, 187; impairment, 7; skills, 187. *See also* Educational achievement; Learning

Acculturating groups: ethnic groups, 25–26, 28–29; immigrants, 25–26, 28–29; native people, 25–26, 28–29; refugees, 25–26, 28–29; sojourners, 25–26, 28–29

Acculturation: attitudes index, 86; definitions of, 20–21, 129–30; modes of, 24, 29; phases of, 29–34; and psychological adaptation, 20, 34, 72–73; resettlement and, 134, 136, 156, 163, 165; and stress, 27–29; torture and, 30

Acting-out behavior, 17, 102, 112, 144, 209

Adaptation, 33–34, 181; acculturation and, 20, 34, 72–73; and assimilation, 23; definition of, 22; physical health and, 72–74; social class and, 70–74; social skills and, 34; social supports and, 72–74; strategies of, 23

Adjustment, 163; academic, 108–10, 112, 122; process of, 176

Adoption, 103, 153

Affective disorder, 156

Alcohol abuse, 94, 96, 101, 196

Alienation, 57, 142

Amerasian children, 149, 153–54, 209

Amnesia, 93, 111

Anger, 8, 13, 141

Anorexia, 143

Antisocial behavior, 104

Anxiety, 58, 134, 208; Cambodian children and, 94, 99, 101; Central American children and, 106, 107, 112; levels of, 116; parental, 12; as a result of community disintegration, 13

Assessment: causes of psychiatric disorder, 130–38; of children's experience, 128–30; data collection, 146–48; psychopathology, 138–45

Assimilationism, 71, 74, 81; and acculturation, 24

Asylum: and phases of acculturation, 31–32; seekers of, 21, 34

Avoidance behavior, 96

Beck Depression Inventory, 95, 96

Behavior modification, 150

Bender Gestalt, 113, 117, 120

Bereavement: outcomes of, 7; risk factors for, 7. *See also* Loss

Biculturalism, 71, 74, 81, 87

Bilingual, bicultural staff, 167, 169–70, 173–74, 184–85, 188, 197. *See also* Cross-cultural teams

Bilingual programs, 108, 167, 169–70, 173–74, 176–78

Boat people, 55, 57

Bulimia, 143

Cambodian adolescents, 8, 9, 138–39, 148, 173, 175, 209, 212–14

Cambodian children, 92–104, 173; and anxiety, 94, 99, 101; and coping, 9, 104; drug abuse by, 94, 101; and foster care, 94, 96; and panic disorders, 94, 100, 101; and post-traumatic stress disorder, 93–101, 104; school adjustment of, 98; and trauma, 92, 93–101, 104; and war and disruption, 94, 96, 100–104

Career development, 185–86, 191

Central American children: adaptive resources, 109, 110; and anxiety, 106, 107, 112; cognitive development of, 120–22;

Author Index

Frederick L. Ahearn, Jr., is dean and professor at the National Catholic School of Social Service of the Catholic University of America, in Washington, D.C. He received a D.S.W. from Columbia University. He is the co-author of *Handbook for Mental Health Care of Disaster Victims* (also from Johns Hopkins) and has written extensively on how ordinary people react to extraordinary, traumatic events. Fluent in Spanish, he has taught in Nicaragua, Chile, and Spain.

Jean L. Athey is Chief, Public Health Social Work, at the federal Maternal and Child Health Bureau. She is responsible for the bureau's violence and unintentional injury prevention program and for working with states in the development of public health social work programs. She received a Ph.D. in Social Services Planning and Administration from the University of Chicago. She served in the Peace Corps and has taught at the University of Oklahoma.

Refugee Children

Designed by Ann Walston

Composed by Brevis Press
in Palatino with Optima display

Printed by The Maple Press Company
on 60-lb. Glatfelter Hi-Brite
and bound in Holliston Roxite